Alternative Therapy
Health Series

Cure Yourself the Natural Way

– in Everyday Life

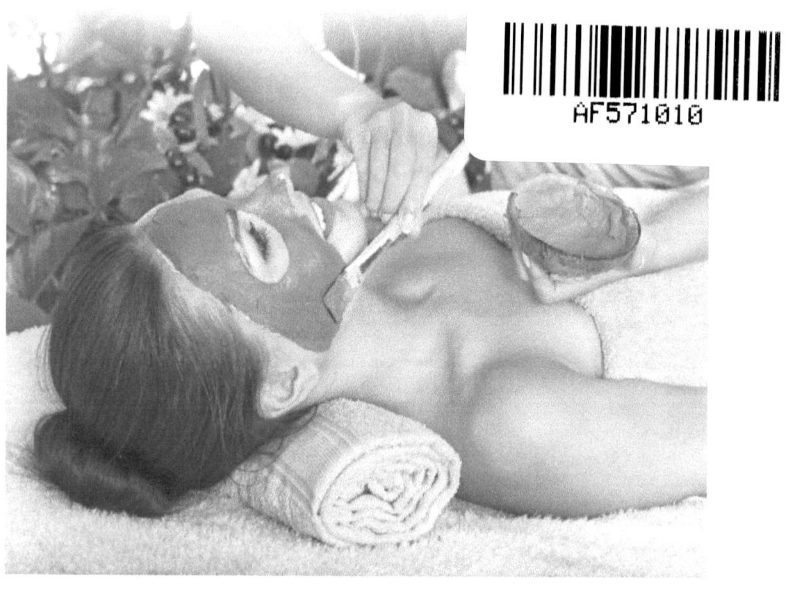

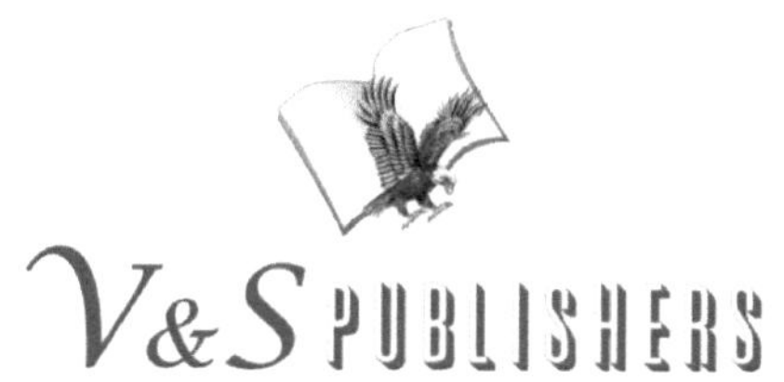

Published by:

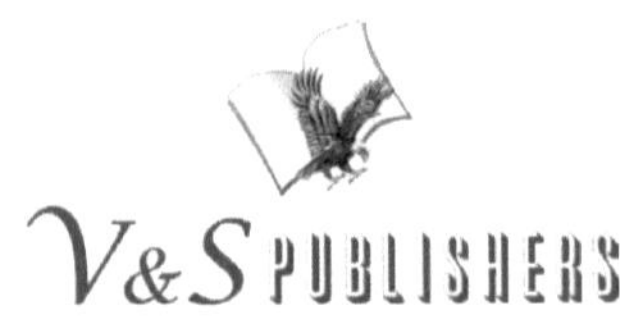

F-2/16, Ansari road, Daryaganj, New Delhi-110002
☎ 23240026, 23240027 • *Fax:* 011-23240028
Email: info@vspublishers.com • *Website:* www.vspublishers.com

Regional Office : Hyderabad
5-1-707/1, Brij Bhawan (Beside Central Bank of India Lane)
Bank Street, Koti, Hyderabad - 500 095
☎ 040-24737290
E-mail: vspublishershyd@gmail.com

Branch Office : Mumbai
Jaywant Industrial Estate, 1st Floor–108, Tardeo Road
Opposite Sobo Central Mall, Mumbai – 400 034
☎ 022-23510736
E-mail: vspublishersmum@gmail.com

ISBN 978-93-579414-5-7

Edition 2020

Publisher's Note

In continuation to our 'Alternative Therapy Health Series', we now come to understand all about Indian Naturopathy. In this form of treatment of disease, Nature's resources-her free gifts-such as fresh air, pure water, bright sunlight, proper and timely sleep, natural diet etc. come into play. Primitive races, before the advent of medical science were utilizing Nature's gifts for the cure of their ailments. The author has tried to prove that how all diseases can be cured and even prevented with Nature's gift made use of in accordance with her own laws and without the help of any drugs. Naturopathy believes that all diseases are due to the accumulation of toxins and waste materials in the human body.

The natural therapy involves application of methods to clear the system from these toxins. The second principle states that due to accumulation of toxins and waste products in the body, various organs get over-exercised causing disharmony in internal body organs and results in growth of germs and diseases. The third principle says that the human body is equipped with a self-healing mechanism, which brings back the body to normal conditions, if proper natural methods are used to assist the system to function correctly.

The book explains the nature's way to cure diseases and ailments through rest, yoga & meditation, fasting, water therapy, mud therapy, aromatherapy, juice therapy, diet therapy, massage therapy, sleep therapy, acupressure etc to recoup the body. Trusted for its no side-effect, treatment by naturopathy as a health care system has gained popularity all over the world. Naturopathic centres have mushroomed in urban areas to restore people's health and well-being.

Kindly treat the below mentioned as a Disclaimer of sorts :

The Editorial Board writes in this book their opinion and that there may be many people who disagree with the conclusions. The publisher and the author, the distributors and bookstores, present this information

Preface

This book grew out to meet the burgeoning need for more professional knowledge about non-mainstream approaches in physical and mental well being. This need to spread awareness has been fueled by the huge consumer-driven trend toward these treatments over the last 2-3 decades. This text aims to provide a reader with cutting edge information from many diverse areas of alternative, complementary, and innovative clinical practice in the area of physical well being and emotional health. The purpose of this work is threefold:

1. To offer a broader, deeper view of information from areas that, although outside mainstream practice, are having an increasing impact and demand.
2. To offer a sense of the level of scientific research and experience associated with complementary and supplementary fields in the area of total health.
3. To further explore and incorporate new treatment options. This text, while not exhaustive, provides a fair overview from the cutting edge of change in health care practices. The overall layout of this 'Alternative Health Care Series' demonstrates the body-mind-spirit premise that permeates diverse field of treatment. By its very nature, this type of book is more focused on divisions and separations--different topics, different sections, and different treatments. Each section begins with a description of the treatment, its safety and/or contraindications, scientific documentation of its efficacy, discussion of which ailment it is best used for, and other important references. Time has come for physicians, clinicians and therapists to have a look at how the marriage of conventional health care to complementary and alternative therapies can offer improved diagnosis than either can alone. The text will offer them more knowledge, a broader viewpoint, and greater option to practice and care for those under their care and attention.

Table of Content's

Indian Naturopathy

Naturopathy, as an age old healing method, was very much in practice in India when drugs and technology were not much in vogue. Nature provided all the elements, within the range of the natural foods, which man needed in the way of nutrient and medicine. Thus, the healing power by naturopathy was nothing new to the Indian tradition. In Indian homes, home remedies have always come before the even doctor's medicines. This clearly portrays the sheer importance of naturopathy as a trustworthy alternative treatment procedure in ancient India. With passing time, Indian naturopathy gained contour as one of the important health care systems in India, famed for its side effect less treatment.

The root of naturopathy as a treatment process is steeped in the antiquities. The origin of naturopathy could be traced right to Vedic period wherein dietary discipline (Pathya and Ahara) and the principles of health (Swastha Vurtha) described in ayurveda have branched out and developed in the form of today's naturopathy. Vedic tradition believed that it is nature, which cures, not the physician and the Vedic culture of ancient India highlighted the use of natures foremost healing agents, water, air, earth and sun which indeed forms the basic crux of naturopathy.

The entire philosophy of naturopathy is thus based upon three basic principles. The first principle of naturopathy believes that all diseases are due to the accumulation of toxins and waste materials in the human body. Thus the therapeutic principle of naturopathy in this case refers to the application of various methods to clear the human system from these toxins and accumulated wastes.

The second principle of naturopathy is again further elaboration of the first principle. According to the second principle when toxins accumulate in the body, the various organs of the body gets over exercised while clearing the toxin off the body. It is when this harmony of internal body organ is disturbed then germs multiply and cause disease. Application of medicine, high dose drugs and vaccines to suppress the symptom of the diseases further aggravates the disease while subduing the symptoms.

The third principle of naturopathy is somewhat a solution of the problems that the first and second principle states. According to the third principle of naturopathy, the human body is equipped with a unique self-healing mechanism, which brings back the body to normal conditions of health, if proper natural methods are used to assist the system to function properly.

The therapeutic practice of naturopathy is based on the principle of naturopathy. Naturopathy believes that the body possesses an inherent ability to "heal thyself"; all the healing powers are within one's body, hence people actually fall ill only when they go against nature. The therapeutic use of naturopathy or the healing power of nature therefore corroborates nearly all the healing techniques in alternative medicine. The basic healing theory of naturopathy is based upon the fact that human being is born healthy and can stay healthy by living in accordance with the laws of nature. To support healthy living and indeed to say no to diseases, Indian naturopathy has described certain nature's way; thus, thorough rest, fasting, water therapy, mud therapy, aromatherapy, message therapy, sleep therapy, acupressure, etc an ailing body can purify and recoup itself

Trusted for its side effect less treatment naturopathy as a health care system has gained importance. The naturopathic centers as the therapeutic centers have mushroomed in large numbers to provide naturopathic treatment especially in the metropolitan cities in India. Most of them follow a similar routine for treating the common ailments. Whether it is the treatment that suits the more spiritually inclined, with yoga and meditation forming an important part of the day's routine, or more modern equipment like saunas and whirlpool baths that take one's fancy, one can choose from many naturopathy centers in India to restore health.

Naturopathy Therapy

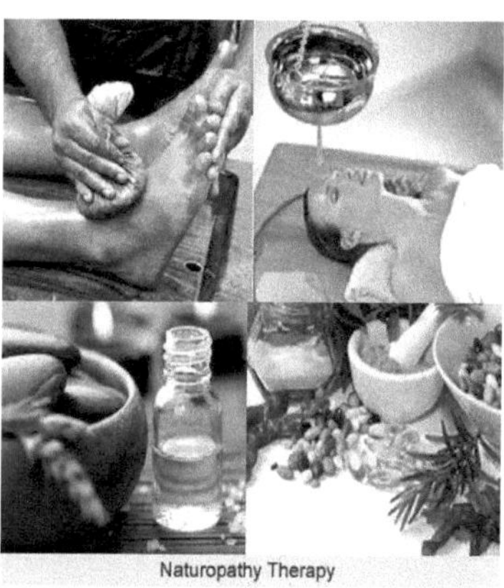
Naturopathy Therapy

Naturopathy Therapy, as an age old healing method, was very much in practice in India when drugs and technology were not much in vogue. Nature provided all the elements, within the range of the natural foods, which man needed in the way of nutrient and medicine. Thus, the healing power by naturopathy was nothing new to the Indian tradition. In Indian homes, home remedies have always come before the even doctor's medicines. This clearly portrays the sheer importance of naturopathy as a trustworthy alternative treatment procedure in ancient India. With passing time, Indian naturopathy gained contour as one of the important health care systems in India, famed for its side effect less treatment.

Raw Juice Therapy

Raw juice therapy which is also known as juice fasting is a method of treatment of ailments through an exclusive diet of juices of fruits and vegetables. This therapy is considered the most effective way to restore health and revitalise the body. In Raw juice therapy, the eliminative and cleansing capacity of the organs of elimination, namely lungs, liver, kidneys and the skin, is greatly increased and masses of accumulated metabolic waste and toxins are quickly removed. Digestion of food and the utilisation of nutrients are greatly improved in this therapy. An exclusive diet of raw juices of fruits and vegetables results in much faster recovery from diseases and more effective cleansing and regeneration of the tissues than the fasting on pure water.

Raw juices of fruits and vegetables are very rich in vitamins, minerals, enzymes and natural sugars. They exercise advantageous effect in normalising all the body functions. They supply needed elements for the body`s own healing activity and cell regeneration, thereby speeding the improvement. Alkaline elements in raw juice is highly beneficial in normalising acid-alkaline balance in the blood and tissues as there is over acidity in most conditions of ill-health. Calcium, potassium and silicon in raw juice help in restoring biochemical and mineral balance in the tissues and cells, thereby preventing premature ageing of cells and disease. Raw juices contain certain natural medicines, vegetal hormones and antibiotics. For instance, string beans are said to contain insulin-like substance.

Sleep Therapy

Sleep therapy in naturopathy is a vital element in man`s mental as well as physical life, since the loss of sleep exerts seriously detrimental effects upon the nervous system. This involves a periodic rest of the body, which is absolutely essential for its efficient functioning.

Abstaining from sleep for longer periods may cause intense psychological changes such as loss of memory, irritability, hallucination and even schizophrenic manifestations. Sleep is the indispensable condition to the recuperation of energy.

Massage Therapy

Massage therapy in Naturopathy is a therapeutic cure to many diseases. It involves the scientific manipulation of the soft tissues of the body. If correctly done on a bare body, it can be highly stimulating and refreshing. Massage therapy dates back as far as 400 B.C., when the great Hippocrates, the father of medicine, employed massage and manipulation in healing his patients. Since then it has been used as a mode of treatment for many ailments and it has restored many a sufferer to health and vigour.

Mud Therapy

Mud therapy has been regarded as an effective remedy to several diseases in ancient times as well as the middle ages. In modern times, it again came into eminence as it was discovered to have remarkable effects to refresh, enliven and vitalise the human body; especially during the night. The forces of earth have remarkable effects upon the human body, especially during the night. It is believed that for wounds and skin diseases, application of clay or moistened earth was the only true natural cure.

Fasting Therapy

Fasting therapy is one of the most ancient customs. This is nature's oldest, most effective and yet least expensive method of treating diseases, recognised as the achievement of natural healing. Throughout medical history, it has been regarded as one of the most dependable curative methods. It refers to complete abstinence from food for a particular period pertaining to a specific purpose. The common cause of all diseases is the accumulation of waste and poisonous matter in the body which results from overeating. The majority of people eats too much and follows sedentary occupations which do not permit sufficient and proper exercise for utilisation of this large quantity of food. This surplus overburdens the digestive organs and clogs up the system with impurities or poisons. Digestion and elimination become slow and the functional activity of the whole system gets deranged. Every disease can be healed by only one remedy - by doing just the opposite of what causes it, that is, by reducing the food intake or fasting. By depriving the body of food for a time ,the organs of elimination such as the bowels, kidneys, skin and lungs are given opportunity to expel, unhampered, the overload of accumulated waste from the system. Thus, fasting therapy is merely the process of purification and an effective and quick method of cure.

Bath Therapy

Bath therapy is a valuable therapeutic agent since time immemorial. In all major ancient civilisations, bathing was considered an important measure for the maintenance of health and prevention of disease. Water has been regarded as an important remedial agent to several diseases such as diarrhoea, ulcerative colitis, fever, jaundice, constipation, and other such ailments. The ancient Vedic literature in India contains numerous references to the efficacy of water in the treatment of disease. There are numerous spas and "Bads" in most European countries where therapeutic baths are used as a major healing agent. Water exerts valuable effects on the human system. It equalises circulation, boosts muscular tone and helps in digestion and nutrition. It also tones up the activity of perspiratory gland and in the process eliminates the damaged cells and toxic matter from the system.

The common water temperature chart is; cold 10 degree Celsius to 18 degree Celsius, neutral 32 degree Celsius to 36 degree Celsius and hot 40 degree Celsius to 45 degree Celsius. Above 45 degree Celsius, water loses its therapeutic value and is destructive. There are several types of Bath therapy which helps in curing gastritis, hyperacidity, indigestion, jaundice, constipation, diarrhoea, dysentery, bronchitis, pleurisy, pneumonia, fever, cough and so on. The various types of bath therapy are enema, cold Ccompress, heating compress, hip bath, spinal bath, full wet sheet pack, cold foot bath, steam bath, immersion bath and Epsom salt bath. These bath therapies are an effective method of cure to several ailments. There are certain methods, duration and process which are to be followed in each therapy.

Diet Therapy

Diet is a very important part of living and a nutritious diet helps keeping new diseases from affecting the body. Ayurveda suggests that only a balanced diet is not sufficient for good health. It recommends that specific bodily conditions require specific diets. It looks at diet as an alternative therapy and treats the body as a combination of three different factors called vata, pitta and kapha. These factors represent air, fire and water respectively. A healthy boy is one in which the three elements are perfectly balanced which can be achieved through diet. When any one of the elements is disturbed the body becomes prone to diseases, correcting the diet can cure it.

Principles of Naturopathy

Naturopathy is a holistic health care system which has its roots deeply seated in the ancient cultural heritage of India. The body has natural abilities to resist diseases and to heal itself- this very concept of naturopathy gains diction amidst the principle of naturopathy.

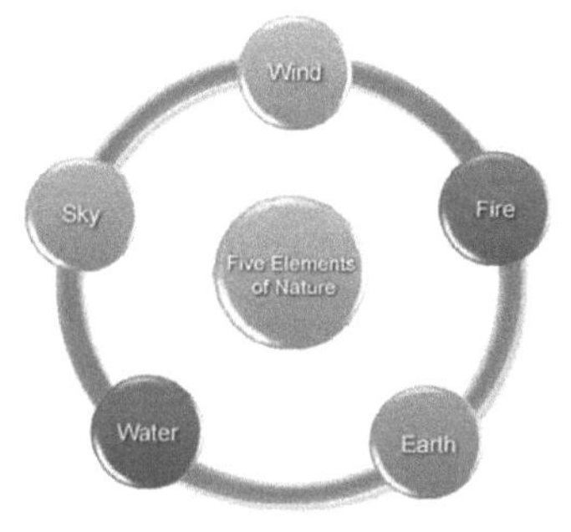

Principles of Naturopathy

Naturopathy believes in the principle of five elements of nature - earth, sky, fire, water, and wind. These five elements form the contour of the naturopathy treatments as these are the source of energy and helps in the treatment. According to the principle of naturopathy therefore, addressing the root cause of ailment and eliminating the root cause is necessary for a healthy body. The principle of naturopathy thus focuses on naturally-occurring and minimally-invasive methods, trusting to the "healing power of nature."

According to the principle of naturopathy, `Pran` is the vitality force. The holistic treatment procedure therefore aims at providing Pran or life force to the body by protecting the body from both the external and internal threats. Although achieving this state is difficult however, it is achievable if and when a harmonious and coordinated functioning of the five elements of nature exists. Naturopathy believes that control over senses is the foundation of good health and therefore a well planned life, sattvic diet and positive thinking is necessary to ensure health.

Naturopathy believes that every human body has germs that grow and multiply and these germs are the source of all sorts of ailment. To prevent germ growth therefore naturopathy prescribes the daily and regular cleaning and detoxification of the body. Naturopathy came as a natural healing process when drugs were not in vogue. Quite ideally therefore the principles of naturopathy do not believe in giving poisonous drugs to kill the germs and to eradicate ailment. Rather naturopathy purifies the blood and tissues to develop immunity, amidst simple nature cure process

The principle of naturopathy is self-described by six core values which are as follows:

- Firstly, naturopathy advises not to harm anybody.
- Naturopathy insist to recognize, respect and promote the self-healing power of nature that underlies in each individual
- Identification and removal of the root causes of illness, rather than eliminating or suppressing symptoms are necessary
- Educating and inspiring rational hope while encouraging self-responsibility for health is needed.
- Naturopathy treats each person by considering all individual health factors and influences.
- Emphasizing the condition of health to promote well-being and to prevent diseases for the individual, each community and indeed the whole world, is one of the basic principles of naturopathy.

Treatment in Naturopathy

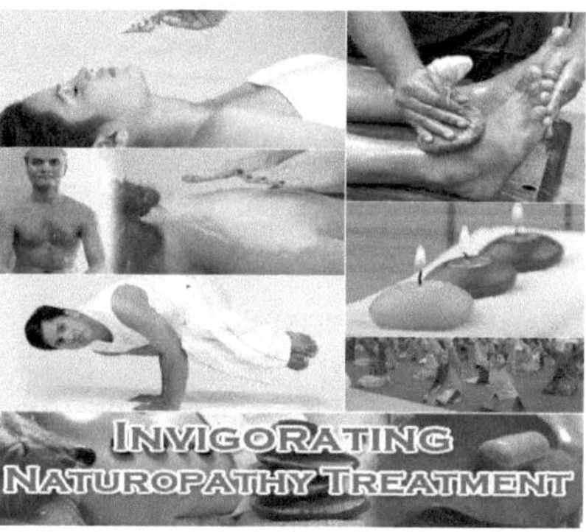

The methods of treatment in naturopathy largely depend on nature and on the process of curing naturally. In India naturopathy treatment is typically a practice of treating diseases by prescribing natural medicines and is completely holistic in nature. Nature can heal all ailments and therefore body can heal naturally -this very concept forms the cornerstone of naturopathy. Thus naturopathy treatment is a form of treatment which emphasizes the tendency of the body to retain a sense of balance and cure itself. Treatments in naturopathy are non toxic and supports in stimulating healing and cleansing responses in a patient.

Treatment in naturopathy involves diagnosis and prescription of modalities and methods of nature. Naturopathic medicines mainly include water, earth, air, light, heat and diet therapy.

Some of the methods of treatment in naturopathy are as follows:

Fasting Therapy: Fasting means complete abstinence from food for a particular period pertaining to a specific purpose and this is nature`s oldest, most effective and yet least expensive method of treating diseases, recognized as the achievement of natural healing. By depriving the body from food for a specific period of time, the organs of elimination such as the bowels, kidneys, skin and lungs are given opportunity to expel, unhampered the overload of accumulated waste from the system. Thus, fasting is merely the process of purification and an effective and quick method of cure, assisting nature in her continuous effort to expel foreign matter and disease producing waste from the body, thereby correcting the faults of improper diet and wrong living.

Mud Therapy : Earth was used extensively for remedial purposes in ancient times as well as the middle ages. In modern times, it again came into prominence as it was discovered to have remarkable effects to refresh, invigorate and vitalize the human body; especially during the night. In the method of treatments in naturopathy it is believed that for wounds and skin diseases, application of clay or moistened earth is the only true natural bandage. Thus, the sleeping or lying on the earth is believed to cure body from several ailments. According to naturopathy mud therapy supports in arousing the entire body from its lethargy to a new manifestation of vital energy. The body then effectively removes old morbid matter and masses of old faeces from the intestines, and receives a sensation of new health, new life and new vigour and strength.

Water Therapy: The largest constituent of human body is water. About 60 to 70 per cent of the total body weight consists of water. Naturopathy recognises the importance of water and the role it plays in human body. Water therapy is therefore an important part in the methods of treatment in naturopathy. Versatility is the most important property of water. According to naturopathy therefore both inside and outside the body water can be effectively used. Liquid, solid or steam any three forms of water can be used according to the need. It can be used hot, cold or lukewarm, for the smooth functioning of all the body processes.

Massage Therapy : According to the methods of treatment in naturopathy an excellent form of passive exercise is massage. A massage involves the scientific manipulation of the soft tissues of the body, which if done correctly, can be highly stimulating and invigorating. Massages have been used from the ancient times, as old as 400 B.C and yet been used as a mode of treatment for many ailments, since it has restored many a sufferer to health and vigour.

Colour Therapy: The method of treatment of diseases by colour is called Chromotherapy. Along with other natural methods of preserving health such as correct diet, adequate rest and relaxation, exercise, yogic asanas and so on it is best used as a supportive therapy. According to practitioners of chromotherapy, the lack of a particular colour in the human system can cause various diseases. Colour therapy in the methods of treatment in naturopathy is a technique of restoring imbalance by means of applying coloured light to the body.

Sleep Therapy: Sleep is one of nature's greatest inventions and blessings of life. It is a periodic rest of the body, which is absolutely essential for its efficient functioning. It has been called "most cheering restorative of tired bodies," since sleep repairs the wear and tear of the body and mind incurred during waking hours. Sleep is thus a vital element in man's mental as well as physical life, since the loss of sleep exerts seriously detrimental effects upon the nervous system. Long periods of wakefulness may cause profound psychological changes such as loss of memory, irritability, hallucination and even schizophrenic manifestations.

Acupressure: In the methods of treatment in naturopathy acupressure is a special form of massage in which fingers or finger-like simple wooden instruments are pressed on certain points of the body to minimize aches, pains, fatigue, tension, stress and various other symptoms of disease. Unlike acupuncture, in which sharp needles are pierced into the points in the skin, Acupressure is non-invasive, safe and simple. In fact, it is a very natural form of physiotherapy, which follows anatomical guides and motor points, stimulation of which relieves various disabilities.

Aromatherapy: Aromatherapy is the alternative branch of medicine that heals and improves the mind and the body, by using natural plant extracts. These plant extract are called essential oils, and are known to convey the "Life Force of Plant". Essential oils can be extracted from the herbs, plants, flowers, fruits, bark, roots or the resin of some trees. These magical extracts from plants can amazingly affect our physical, mental, emotional and even spiritual being. Whether it's beautifying the skin, reducing weight, prevention and cure of diseases, inducing sexual attraction, relieving tension and anxiety, to sedate or refresh individuals, the essential oils come in handy.

Magnetic Therapy: Magnetic healing is a science as well as an art demanding knowledge of human organism and the skill to cure through proper application of magnets. In the methods of treatment in naturopathy magnets are designed specially for human applications as magnets have the power to interact with the energy system of the body, to create a different field for efficient cellular and hence organic activities. Magnets are applied to a painful area of the body to stimulate the nerves in that area for pain relief, as a part of the nature's healing process.

Exercises in Naturopathy

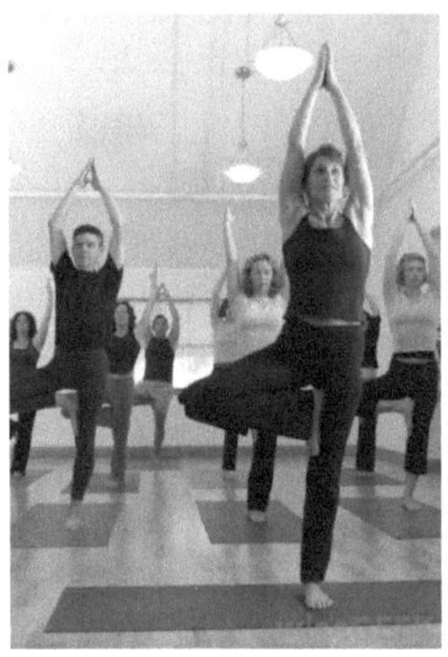

Exercise in Naturopathy is essential for the maintenance of normal condition of life. Lack of natural exercise is one of the principal causes of weakness and ill health. In recent years, the requirement for exercise has been recognised even in sickness. Exercises are now standard procedures in medicine to refurbish the use of muscles and nerves that have been injured by disease or by accident.

Exercise and Activity

It is vital to make a distinction between exercise and activity. While both are imperative as they are involved in essential physical movement, they differ in degree and benefits. Both make use of the body in voluntary movement. Activity uses the body to a limited degree and normally to achieve a specific purpose. Exercise employs the body over the widest possible range of movement for the particular purpose of maintaining or acquiring muscle tone and control with maximum joint flexibility. Activity requires less physical effort and often less conscious effort once the routine has been established. Exercise demands substantial physical effort and is more advantageous as mental concentration is simultaneously employed.

Methods of Exercise

A number of systems of exercise have been developed over the years, the most well-liked among them being the Swedish system and yoga asanas, the later having been practised from ancient times in India. Whichever system one may choose to take on, the exercises should be performed methodically, on a regular basis and under proper guidance. To be really functional, exercise should be taken in such a manner as to bring into action all the muscles of the body in a natural way. Walking is one such exercise. It is, however, so gentle in character that one must walk several kilometers in a brisk manner to add up to a fair amount of exercise. Other forms of good exercise are swimming, cycling, horse riding, tennis, etc.

Benefits of Exercise

Regular exercise taken appropriately can achieve the increased use of food by the body, which contributes to health and fitness. The basal metabolic rate and habitual body temperature will gradually rise during several weeks of physical exercise, if the programme is not too hard. The healthy person more often than not has abundant body heat and a warm radiant glow. Progressive physical exercise on a regular basis can bring about the balance of automatic, or involuntary, nervous system. Exercise can prevent or lessen gravitational ptosis or sag, as it is commonly called. Improved capillary action in the working of muscular and brain tissue results from exercise carried to the point of real endurance. This permits greater blood flow and gives the muscles, including the heart, more resistance to fatigue. The full use of the lungs in vigorous exercise can reduce or prevent lung congestion due to lymph accumulation. Better respiratory reserve is developed by persistent exercise. This ensures better breath holding, particularly after a standard exercise. With greater respiratory reserves, exercises become easier. Consistent exercise leads to improvement in quality of blood. Systemic exercise promotes physical strength and mental vigour and strengthens will power and self control leading to pleasant development of the whole system.

Precautions in Exercise

Dynamic exercise of any kind should not be taken for an hour and a half after eating, or straight away before meals. Weak patients and those suffering from serious diseases like cancer, heart trouble, tuberculosis and asthma should not undertake vigorous exercise except under the supervision of an experienced physician. If exercising makes one tired, then he should stop immediately. The purpose of exercise should be to make one feel refreshed and relaxed and not exhausted. The most important rule about the fitness plan is to start with very light exercise and to increase the effort in gradual and easy stages. The sense of well being will begin almost immediately.

Importance of Amino Acids in Naturopathy

In Naturopathy there is immense importance of Amino Acids. Proteins are exceptionally complex organic compounds of the elements hydrogen, oxygen, carbon, nitrogen, and with some exceptions, sulphur. Each type contains a definite number of building blocks known as amino acids. When food stuffs are ingested, the nutrients and amino acids do not immediately disseminate into all the different tissues. There are a series of biochemical reactions in the digestive tract which collect these proteins, break them down and then utilise them as needed. There are about twenty two amino acids needed for the normal functioning of the body. The body can manufacture many amino acids if it has no sufficient nitrogen source, but it cannot produce certain others in adequate amounts to meet its needs.

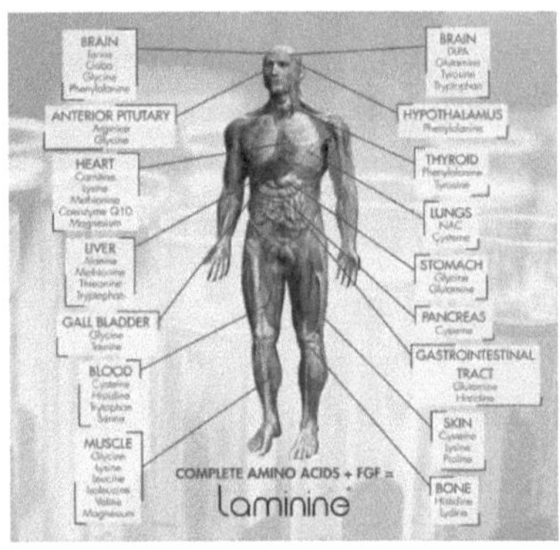

Much research has been done on amino acids in recent times and this has paved the way for dramatic cure and treatment of different problems by their judicious use. The various functions of the necessary and regularly investigated non essential amino acids, their deficiency symptoms and their therapeutic uses are discussed below:

Tryptophan

Of all the vital amino acids, tryptophan is the one that is most investigated by nutrition researchers. It is essential to blood clotting, digestive juices and the optic system. It induces sleep and quietens the nervous system. It wards off signs of premature old age; cataracts of the eyes, baldness, and weakening of sex glands and deformity of teeth enamel. It is also essential to the female reproductive organs and for appropriate utilisation of vitamin A by the body. Major sources of this amino acid are nuts, and most vegetables. Lack of tryptophan causes symptoms similar to those of vitamin A deficit. A number of scientists feel that it can be used as a harmless and effective food remedy for insomnia Tryptophan as a food medicine should be taken between meals with a low protein food such as fruit juice or bread.

Methionine

This is very important sulphur -bearing compound which helps dissolve cholesterol and assimilates fat. It is required by haemoglobin, the pancreas, the lymph and the spleen. It is necessary to maintain normal body weight and also helps maintain the proper nitrogen balance in the body. Rich sources of methionine are Brazil nut, hazal nut, and other nuts. It is also found in cauliflower, pineapples, brussel sprouts, cabbage, and apples. Its insufficiency can lead to chronic rheumatic fever in children, cirrhosis and nephritis of the kidneys. Studies show that methionine and chorine thwart tumours and proliferation.

Lysine

Lysine inhibits viruses. Its use along with vitamin C, zinc and vitamin A helps get rid of virus infections. Vitamin C protects this amino acid while in the body so that lysine plus vitamin C has a much stronger anti-virus effect than if either is used separately. Lysine also influences the female reproductive cycle. Lack of sufficient lysine in the diet may cause dizziness, nausea, headaches, and incipient anaemia. The main sources of this amino acid are most kinds of nuts, seeds, vegetables and sub-acid fruits. Lysine upsets in the body have also been associated with pneumonia, nephritis and acidosis as well as malnutrition and rickets in children.

Valine

Valine is an indispensable body growth factor, chiefly for mammary glands and ovaries. Valine is directly linked with the nervous system. It is necessary for the prevention of nervous and digestive disorders. Major sources are almonds, apples and most vegetables. Lack of this amino acid makes a person sensitive to touch and sound.

Isoleucine

This amino acid is vital for maintaining the nitrogen balance fundamental to all body functions. It also regulates metabolism of the thymus, spleen and pituitary glands. Rich sources are sunflower seeds, all nuts, except cashew nuts, avacados and olives.

Leucine

It is the compliment of isoleucine, with a similar chemical composition although in different arrangement. Its functions and sources are also the same.

Phenylalanine

This is indispensable to the production of hormone adrenaline; to the production of the thyroid secretion and the hair and skin pigment, melanin. It is useful in weight control because of its effect on the thyroid. Its use before meals suppresses the appetite to a large extent. It is necessary for the efficient functioning of kidneys and bladder. Major source are nuts, parsley, seeds, carrots and tomatoes. An important recently discovered restorative use of phenylalanine is its capacity to overcome most conditions of lethargy through stimulation of adrenaline.

Threonine

This amino acid is found in various types of milk and is a major constituent in cow`s milk. Other sources are seeds, carrots, nuts, and green vegetables. Without threonine, a child`s development will be deficient and there will be malfunctioning of the brain. This amino acid has a dominant anti convulsive effect.

Histidine

This helps tissue development and repair. It is active in producing normal blood supply. It is also vital to the formation of glycogen in the liver. It is found in the root vegetables and all green vegetables. Studies show that the free form of histidine in the blood is low in cases of rheumatoid arthritis and if taken orally, may possibly slow down the symptoms of this illness. Oral histidine has, however, a propensity to stimulate hydrochloric acid secretion in the stomach and persons who are vulnerable to an overabundance of acid and also those who have ulcers should keep away from taking pure histidine. Orthopaedic and joint pains are caused by lack of histidine.

Arginine

This is called the "fatherhood "amino acid as it comprises 80 per cent of all male reproductive cells. It is crucial for normal growth. Serious lack of this amino acid reduces the sex instinct causing impotence. It is found in most vegetables, in particular, green and root vegetables.

Cystine

It provides resistance by building up white cell activity. It is an indispensable amino acid. It is one of the mainstays of health as it is necessary for the proper formation of skin and helps one recover from surgery. It is used in the healing of skin diseases, for low white blood cells counts and for some cases of anaemia.

Tyrosine

This can be called an anti-stress amino acid. Tyrosine is also advantageous for nervousness, irritability, depression and despondency. Research has established this amino acid to be effectual in the management and control of depression in conjunction with glutamine, tryptophan, niacin and vitamin B6. It is also useful in the treatment of allergies and high blood pressure. When tyrosine is taken, a supplement of Valine, another important amino acid should not be taken as Valine may block tyrosine`s entry to the brain.

Glutamine

This little known non-essential amino acid is considered valuable in the treatment of alcoholism. Glutamine reduces the generally irresistible craving for alcohol that recovering drinkers almost inevitably encounter.

When one or more of the fundamental amino acids are left out of the diet, symptoms similar to those of vitamin deficiencies may be experienced such as low blood pressure, loss of weight, poor resistance to infections, anaemia, poor muscle tone, slow healing of wounds and bloodshot eyes. Children who do not get the requisite amounts of amino acids in their every day diet suffer from stunted growth and lasting damage to the glands. On the other hand, those getting the full proportion of amino acids in their diet will be rewarded with vigour, energy and long life. The best food proteins with all the important amino acids are found in almonds, cheese and eggs. Amino acids are being increasingly and effectively used in the treatment of several diseases, such as stomach ulcers, burns, kidney diseases and liver diseases. It has also been observed that the diseases of old age can be largely prevented if elderly persons take the proper food supplements of amino acids, vitamins and minerals. Amino acids are required at every stage from infancy to old age, to repair worn out tissues and to create new ones.

Enzymes in Naturopathy

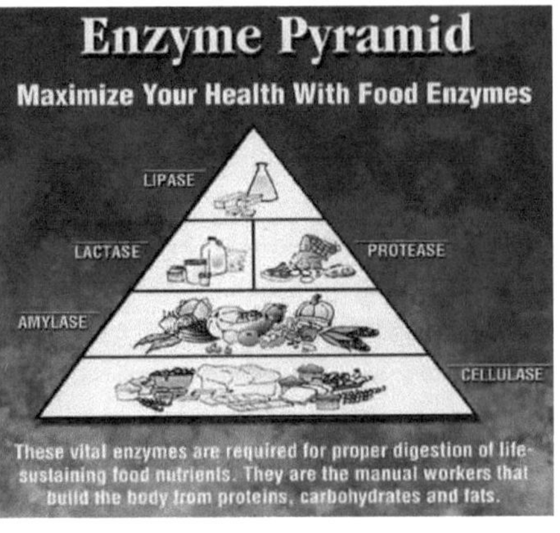

Enzymes in Naturopathy are of enormous importance. Enzymes are chemical substances produced in the living organism. Enzymes are part of all living cells, including those of plants and animals. Although enzymes are produced in the living cell, they are not dependent upon the fundamental processes of the cell and work outside the cell. Certain enzymes of yeast, for example, when expressed from the yeast cells are competent of exerting their usual effect, that is, the conversion of sugar to alcohol. A prominent feature of enzymes is that while they enter into chemical reaction, they stay intact in the process.

Enzymes are protein molecules made up of chains of amino acids. They play a very important role and work more capably than any reagent concocted by chemists. The specificity of an enzyme is related to the formation of the enzyme substrate complex which requires that the proper groupings of both substrate and enzyme should be in correct relative position. Enzymes which are used in the cells which make them are called intracellular enzymes. Enzymes which are produced in cells which secrete them to other parts of the body are known as extra cellular enzymes. Digestive juices are an instance of the latter type. There are few enzymes, whose names have been established by long usage such as ptyalin, pepsin, trypsin and erepsin. Apart from these, enzymes are generally named by adding the suffixes to the main part of the name of the substrate upon which they act. Thus amylases act upon starch (amylum), lactase acts upon lactose, lipases act upon lipids, maltase acts upon maltose and protesses act upon lipids, maltase acts upon maltose and protesses act upon proteins.

There are, nevertheless, quite a lot of enzymes which act upon many substances in different ways. These enzymes are named by their functions rather than substrates. Some enzymes work proficiently only if some other specific substance is present in addition to substrate. This other substance is known as an “activator” or a “conenzyme”. Many of the conenzymes are related to vitamins. Conenzymes, like enzymes, are being incessantly regenerated in the cells. Enzymes play a crucial role in the digestion of food as they are responsible for the chemical changes which the food undergoes for the period of digestion. The chemical changes comprise the breaking up of the large molecules of carbohydrates, fats and proteins into smaller ones or conversion of complex substances into simple ones which can be absorbed by the intestines.

Enzymes also control the numerous reactions by which these simple substances are utilised in the body for building up new tissues and producing energy. The enzymes themselves are not broken down or changed in the process. They remain as powerful at the end of a reaction as they were at the beginning. Furthermore, very small amounts can convert large amounts of material. They are thus true catalysts. The process of digestion begins in the mouth. The saliva in the mouth, besides helping to masticate the food, carries an enzyme called ptyalin which begins the chemical action of digestion. It initiates the catabolism of carbohydrates by converting starches into simple sugars. This explains the need for systematic mastication of starchy food in the mouth. If this is not done the ptyalin cannot carry out its functions as it is active in an alkaline, neutral or slightly acid medium and is inactivated by the extremely acid gastric juices in the stomach. Even though enzymatic action starts while food is being chewed, digestion moves into high gear only when the chewed food has passed the esophagus and reached the stomach. The enzyme or active principle of the gastric juice is pepsin. This enzyme in combination with hydrochloric acid starts the breakdown of proteins into absorbable amino acids called polypeptides. An additional enzyme, rennin, plays an imperative role in the stomach of the infant.

The pancreas contributes various enzymes which carry on the breakdown of proteins, help to divide starch into sugars and work with bile in digesting fats. The small intestine itself secretes enzymes from its inner wall to complete the reactions. When all the enzymes have done their work, the food is digested and rendered fit for absorption by the system. Raw foods contain enzymes in abundance; pasteurising, pickling, cooking, smoking and other processing denature enzymes. It is, therefore, necessary to include in our diet, considerable amount of raw foods in the form of fruits, raw salads and sprouts. Studies have revealed that the body without sufficient raw materials from raw foods may exhaust and produce fewer enzymes year after year. This may lead to wearing out of body processes and consequent worn out looks.

Importance of Vitamins in Naturopathy

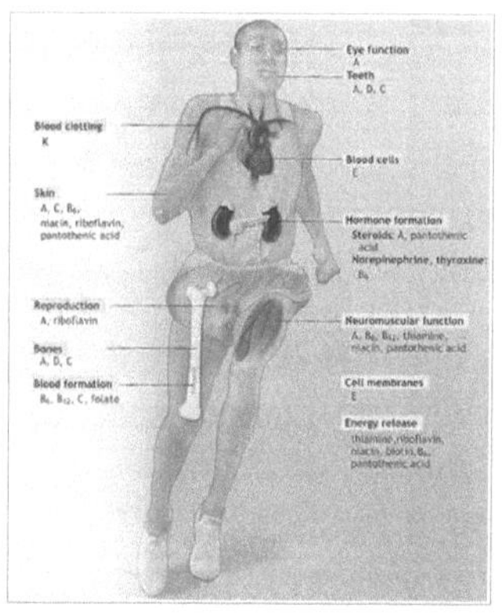

Vitamine` meaning a vital amine, is of great importance in Naturopathy. Vitamins are potent organic compounds which are found in small concentrations in foods and perform specific and vital functions in the body chemistry. Except for a few exceptions, they cannot be manufactured or synthesised by the organism and their absence or improper absorption results in specific deficiency disease. It is not possible to sustain life without all the essential vitamins. In their natural state they are found in minute quantities in organic foods. Vitamins, which are of several kinds, differ from each other in physiological function, in chemical structure and in their distribution in food.

Vitamins are broadly divided into two categories, namely, fat-soluble and water-soluble. Vitamins A, D, E and K are all soluble in fat and fat solvents and are therefore, known as fat-soluble. They are not easily lost by ordinary cooking methods and they can be stored in the body to some extent, mostly in the liver. They are measured in international units. Vitamin B Complex and C are water soluble. They are dissolved easily in cooking water. A portion of these vitamins may actually be destroyed by heating. They cannot be stored in body and hence they have to be taken daily in foods. Any extra quantity taken in any one day is eliminated as waste.

The various functions of common vitamins, their deficiency symptoms, natural sources, daily requirements and their therapeutic uses are discussed in brief as follows:

Vitamin A

Known as anti-opathalmic, vitamin A is essential for growth and vitality. It builds up resistance to respiratory and other infections and works mainly on the eyes, lungs, stomach and intestines. It prevents eye diseases and plays a vital role in nourishing the skin and hair. It helps to prevent premature ageing, increases life expectancy and extends youthfulness. The main sources of this vitamin are fish liver oil, liver, whole milk, curds, pure ghee, butter, cheese, cream and egg yolk, green leafy and certain yellow root vegetables such as spinach, lettuce, turnip, carrot, cabbage and tomato and ripe fruits such as prunes, mangoes, papaya, apricots, peaches, almonds and other dry fruits. A prolonged deficiency of vitamin A may result in inflammation of the eyes, poor vision frequent colds, night blindness and increased susceptibility to infections, lack of appetite and vigour, defective teeth and gums and skin disorders.

Vitamin B Complex

There are a large variety of vitamins in the B group, the more important being B1 or thiamine, B2 or riboflavin, B3 or niacin or nicotinic acid, B6 or pyridoxine, B9 or folic acid, B12 and B5 or pantothenic acid. B vitamins are synergistic. They are more potent together than when used separately.

Thiamine

Known as anti-neuritic and anti-ageing vitamin, thiamine plays an important role in the normal functioning of the nervous system, the regulation of carbohydrates and good digestion. It protects heart muscle, stimulates brain action and helps prevent constipation. It has a mild diuretic effect. Valuable sources of this vitamin are wheat germ, yeast, the outer layer of whole grains, cereals, pulses, nuts, peas, legumes, dark green leafy vegetables, milk, egg, banana and apple. The deficiency of thiamine can cause serious impairment of the digestive system and chronic constipation, loss of weight, diabetes, mental depression, nervous exhaustion and weakness of the heart.

Riboflavin

Vitamin B2 or riboflavin, also known as vitamin G, is essential for growth and general health as also for healthy eyes, skin, nails and hair. It helps eliminate sore mouth, lips and tongue. It also functions with other substances to metabolise carbohydrates, fats, and protein. The main sources of this vitamin are green leafy vegetables, milk, cheese, wheat germ, egg, almonds, sunflower, seeds, citrus fruits and tomatoes.

Its deficiency can cause a burning sensation in the legs, lips and tongue, oily skin, premature wrinkles on face and arm and eczema.

Niacin

Vitamin B3 or niacin or nicotinic acid is essential for proper circulation, healthy functioning of the nervous system and proper protein and carbohydrate metabolism. It is essential for synthesis of sex hormones, thyroxin and insulin. It is contained in liver, fish, and poultry, peanut, whole wheat, green leafy vegetables, dates, figs, prunes and tomato. A deficiency can lead to skin eruptions, frequent stools, mental depression, insomnia, chronic headaches, digestives disorders and anaemia.

Pyridoxine

Vitamin B6 or pyridoxine is actually a group of substance: pyridoxine, pyridoxinal and pyridoxamine that are closely related and function together. It helps in the absorption of fats and proteins, prevents nervous and skin disorders and protects against degenerative diseases. The main sources of this vitamin are yeast, wheat, bran, wheat germ, pulses, cereals, banana, walnuts, milk, egg, liver, meat and fresh vegetables. Deficiency can lead to dermatitis, conjunctivitis, anaemia, depression, skin disorders, nervousness, insomnia, migraine headaches and heart diseases.

Folic Acid

Vitamin B9 or folic acid, along with vitamin B12 is necessary for the formation of red blood cells. It is essential for the growth and division of all body cells for healing processes. It aids protein metabolism and helps prevent premature greying. Valuable sources of this vitamin are deep green leafy vegetables such as spinach, lettuce, brewers yeast, mushrooms, nuts, peanuts and liver. A deficiency can result in certain types of anaemia, serious skin disorders, and loss of hair, impaired circulation, fatigue and mental depression.

Pantothenic Acid

Vitamin B5 or pantothenic acid helps in cell building, maintaining normal growth and development of the central nervous system. It stimulates the adrenal glands and increases the production of cortisone and other adrenal hormones. It is essential for conversion of fatty and sugar to energy. It also helps guard against most physical and mental stresses and toxins and increases vitality. The main sources of this vitamin are whole grain bread and cereals, green vegetables, peas, beans, peanuts and egg yolk. It can be synthesised in the body by intestinal bacteria. A deficiency can cause chronic fatigue, hypoglycaemia, greying and loss of hair, mental depression, stomach disorders, and blood and skin disorders.

Vitamin B12

Vitamin B_{12} or cobalamin, commonly known as red vitamin, is the only vitamin that contains essential mineral elements. It is essential for proper functioning of the central nervous system, production and regeneration of red blood cells and proper utilisation of fat, carbohydrates and protein for body building. It also improves concentration, memory and balance. Valuable sources of this vitamin are kidney, liver, meat, milk, eggs, bananas and peanuts. Its deficiency can lead to certain types of anaemia, poor appetite and loss of energy and mental disorders.

Vitamin C

Vitamin C or ascorbic acid is essential for normal growth and the maintenance of practically all the body tissues, especially those of the joints, bones, teeth, and gums. It protects one against infections and acts as a harmless antibiotic. It promotes healing and serves as protection against all forms of stress and harmful effects of toxic chemicals. It helps prevent and cure the common cold. It also helps in decreasing blood cholesterol. This vitamin is found in citrus fruits, berries, green and leafy vegetables, tomatoes, potatoes, and green grams. A deficiency can cause scurvy marked by weakness, anaemia, bleeding gums and painful and swollen parts, slow healing of sores and wounds, premature ageing and lowered resistance to all infections.

Vitamin D

Vitamin D is necessary for proper bone and teeth formation and for the healthy functioning of the thyroid gland. It assists in the assimilation of calcium, phosphorus and other minerals from the digestive tract. This vitamin is found in the rays of the sun, fish, milk, eggs, butter and sprouted seeds. A deficiency can cause gross deformation of bones and severe tooth decay.

Vitamin E

Vitamin E is essential for normal reproductory functions, fertility and physical vigour. It prevents unsaturated fatty acids, sex hormones and fat soluble vitamins from being destroyed in the body by oxygen. It dilutes blood vessels and improves circulation. It is essential for the prevention of heart diseases, asthma, arthritis, and many other conditions. It is available in wheat or cereals germ, whole grain products, green leafy vegetables, milk, eggs, all whole, raw or sprouted seeds and nuts. Its deficiency can lead to sterility in men and repeated abortions in women, degenerative developments in the coronary system, strokes and heart disease.

Vitamin K

Vitamin K is necessary for the proper clotting of blood, prevention of bleeding and normal liver functions. It aids in reducing excessive menstrual flow. This vitamin is contained in egg yolk, cow's milk, yogurt, alfalfa, green and leafy vegetables, spinach, cauliflower, cabbage and tomato. Its deficiency can lead to sufficient bile salts in the intestines, colitis, lowered vitality and premature ageing.

Importance of Minerals in Naturopathy

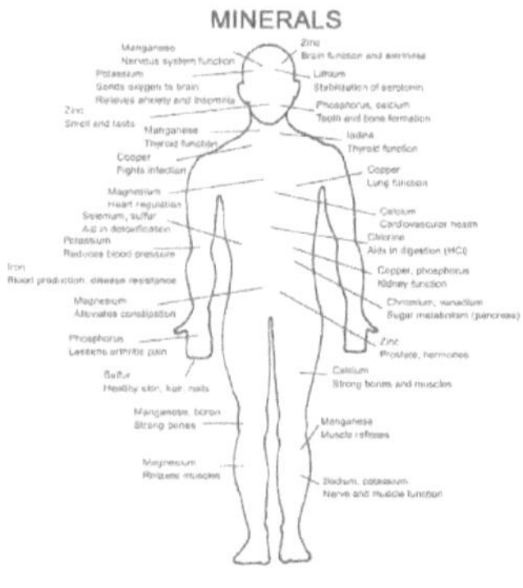

Minerals are of immense importance in naturopathy. Like vitamins and amino acids minerals are crucial for regulating and building the trillions of living cells which make up the body. Body cells receive the vital food elements through the blood stream. They must, therefore, be appropriately nourished with an adequate supply of all the essential minerals for the well organised functioning of the body. Minerals help maintain the volume of water necessary to life processes in the body. They help draw chemical substances into and out of the cells and they keep the blood and tissue fluid from becoming either too acidic or too alkaline. The mineral elements which are needed by the body in substantial amounts are sulphur, magnesium, calcium, phosphorous, iron, sodium, potassium and chlorine. In addition the body needs minute amounts of iodine, manganese, zinc, copper, cobalt, selenium, silicon, fluorine and some others.

Calcium

The human body needs calcium more than any other mineral. Calcium performs many essential functions. Without this mineral, the contractions of the heart would be defective, the muscles would not contract correctly to make the limbs move and blood would not clot. Calcium stimulates enzymes in the digestive process and coordinates the functions of all other minerals in the body. Calcium is found in milk and milk products, whole wheat, leafy vegetables such as carrots, lemons, lettuce, watercress, oranges, spinach, and cabbage, almonds, figs and walnuts. Deficit may cause porous and fragile bones, insomnia, tooth decay, muscle cramps, heart palpitations, and irritability. Liberal quantity of calcium is also required when excessive calcium has been lost from the body as in hyperparathyroidism or chronic renal disease.

Phosphorus

This mineral combines with calcium to create the calcium -phosphorus balance required for the growth of bones and teeth and in the formation of nerve cells. Phosphorus is also important for the assimilation of carbohydrates and fats. It is a stimulant to the nerves and brain. Phosphorous is found in abundance in nuts, egg yolk, fruit juices, cereals, pulses, milk and legumes. Usually about one gram of phosphorous is considered necessary in the daily diet. A phosphorous shortage may bring about loss of weight, reduced sexual powers, retarded growth, and weakness.

Iron

Iron is a significant mineral which enters into the vital activity of the blood and glands. Iron exists for the most part as haemoglobin in the blood. It distributes the oxygen inhaled into the lungs to all the cells. It is the master mineral which creates warms, vivacity and stamina. It is necessary for the healthy complexion and for building up resistance in the body. The chief sources of iron are whole grain, cereals, dried beans, grapes, raisins, spinach, all green vegetables, dark coloured fruits, beets, dates, liver and egg yolk. Iron deficiency is in general caused by severe blood loss, malnutrition, infections and by excessive use of drugs and chemicals. Iron is the classic medication for anaemia.

Sulphur

All living matter contains some sulphur; this element is as a result essential for life. The main function of sulphur is to dissolve waste materials. It helps to eject some of the waste and poisons from the system. It helps keep the skin clear of blemishes and makes hair glossy. It is also important in rheumatic conditions. The main sulphur containing foods are cabbage, cheese, dried beans, radishes, carrots, fish and eggs. Deficiency of sulphur may cause eczema and imperfect development of hair and nails. Sulphur creams and ointments have been outstandingly successful in treating a variety of skin problems.

Magnesium

All human tissues contain little amounts of magnesium. Next to potassium, magnesium is the chief metallic action in living cells. Magnesium helps one keep calm and cool during the sweltering summer months. It aids in keeping nerves relaxed and generally balanced. It is essential for all muscular activity. This mineral is in activator for most of the enzyme system involving carbohydrate, fat and protein in energy producing reactions. Magnesium helps prevent calcium deposits in kidneys and gallstones and also brings relief from indigestion. Magnesium is widely distributed in nuts, almonds, whole grains, soyabeans, lemons, peaches, brown rice, alfalfa, apples, figs, sunflower seeds and sesame seeds. Deficiency can lead to heart attack, epileptic seizures, nervous irritability, kidney damage and kidney stones, muscle cramps, arteriosclerosis, marked depression and confusion, impaired protein metabolism and premature wrinkles.

Sodium

Sodium Chloride, the chemical name for common salt, contains 39 per cent of sodium, an element which never occurs in free form in nature. It is found in an associated form with many minerals particularly in plentiful amounts with chlorine. It acts with other electrolytes, mainly potassium, in the intracellular fluid, to control the osmotic pressure and maintain an appropriate water balance within the body. Sodium can help prevent catarrh. It promotes a clear brain, resulting in a better disposition and less mental exhaustion. Vegetable foods rich in sodium are celery, cucumbers, beet-tops, cabbage, lettuce, watermelon, lemons, oranges, grapefruit, corn, lady`s fingers, apple, berries, pears, squash, pumpkin, peaches, lentils, almonds and walnuts. Animal food sources include lean beef, kidney, shell fish, bacon and cheese. Deficiencies of sodium are, however, rare and may be caused by excessive sweating, prolonged use of diuretics, or chronic diarrhoea. Deficiency may lead to muscular weakness, heat exhaustion, nausea, mental apathy and respiratory failure.

Potassium

Potassium is indispensable to the life of every cell of a living being and is among the most liberally and widely distributed of all the tissue minerals. It is found predominantly in the intracellular fluid where it plays an important role as a catalyst in energy metabolism and in the synthesis of glycogen and protein. Potassium is necessary for muscle contraction and therefore, important for appropriate heart function. It promotes the secretion of hormones and helps the kidneys in detoxification of blood. Potassium prevents female disorders by stimulating the endocrine hormone production. It is involved in the proper execution of the nervous system and helps overcome weariness. It also aids in clear thinking by sending oxygen to the brain and assists in reducing blood pressure. Potassium is widely distributed in foods. All vegetables, especially green, leafy vegetables, whole grains, lentils, sunflower seeds, nuts, grapes, oranges, lemons, raisins, milk, cottage cheese and butter milk are rich sources. Potassium deficiency may occur during gastrotestinal disturbances with severe vomiting and diarrhoea, diabetic acidosis and potassium losing nephritis. In simple cases of potassium deficiency, drinking plenty of tender coconut water on a daily basis can make up for it.

Chlorine

In the human body, chlorine is liberated by the interaction of common salt, taken along with food, and hydrochloric acid liberated in the stomach during the process of digestion. It is important for the proper distribution of carbon dioxide and the maintenance of osmotic pressure in the tissues. Chlorine regulates the blood`s alkaline acid balance and works with Potassium in a compound form. It aids in the cleaning out of body waste by helping the liver to function. Chlorine is found in cheese and other milk products, rice, radishes, lentils, coconuts, green leafy vegetables, tomatoes, all berries, and egg yolk. Deficiency of this mineral can cause loss of hair and teeth.

Iodine

The chief store house of iodine in the body is the thyroid gland. Iodine regulates the rate of energy production and body weight and promotes proper growth. It improves mental alacrity and promotes healthy nails, skin, hair and teeth. The best dietary sources of iodine are kelp and other seaweeds. Other good sources are pineapples, pears, artichokes, citrus fruits, turnip greens, garlic, watercress, egg yolk and seafood and fish liver oils. Small doses of iodine are of great value in the prevention of goitre in areas where it is endemic and are of value in treatments, at least in the early stages.

Copper

There are approximately 75 to 150 mg. of copper in the adult human body. Newborn infants have higher concentrations than adults. This mineral helps in the conversion of iron into haemoglobin. It stimulates the growth of red blood cells. It is also a fundamental part of certain digestive enzymes. It makes the amino acid tyrosine usable, enabling it to work as the pigmenting factor for hair and skin. It is also necessary for the utilisation of vitamin C. Copper is found in most foods containing iron, particularly in almonds, peas, lentils, whole wheat, dried beans, prunes and egg yolk. A copper insufficiency may result in bodily weakness, digestive disturbances and impaired respiration.

Cobalt

Cobalt is a component of vitamin B12, a nutritional factor required for the formation of red blood cells. The presence of this mineral in foods helps the synthesis of haemoglobin and the absorption of food- iron. The best dietary sources of cobalt are meat, kidney and liver. All green leafy vegetables contain some amount of this mineral.

Manganese

The human body contains 30 to 35 mg. of manganese, widely distributed throughout the tissues. It is found in the pancreas, kidney, liver, pituitary glands. This mineral helps nurture the nerves and brain and aids in the coordination of nerve impulses and muscular actions. It helps get rid of fatigue and reduces nervous irritability. Manganese is found in citrus fruits, the outer covering of nuts, grains, in the green leaves of edible plants, fish and raw egg yolk. A deficiency of this mineral can lead to poor elasticity in the muscles, confused thinking, dizziness, and poor memory.

Zinc

There are about two grams of zinc in the body where it is extremely concentrated in the eyes, nails, hair, skin and testes. Zinc is a precious mineral. It is needed for healthy skin and hair, proper healing of wounds, successful pregnancies and male virility. It plays a vital role in guarding against diseases and infection. The main dietary sources of zinc are beans, meat, whole grains, milk, liver, nuts, and seeds. Deficiency can result in weight loss, skin diseases, and loss of hair, poor appetite, diarrhoea and frequent infection. Those suffering from rheumatoid arthritis may have a zinc deficit.

Selenium

Selenium and vitamin E are synergistic and the two together are stronger than the sum of the equal parts. Selenium slows down ageing and hardening of tissues through oxidation. Selenium is useful in keeping youthful elasticity in tissues. It alleviates hot flushes and menopausal distress. It also helps in the prevention and treatment of dandruff. This mineral is found in Brewer`s yeast, garlic, onions, tomatoes, eggs, milk and sea food. Deficiency of this mineral can cause premature loss of stamina.

Silicon

Silicon is indispensable for the growth of skin, hair shafts, nails and other outer coverings of the body. It also makes the eyes bright and helps in hardening the enamel of the teeth. It is advantageous in all healing process and protects body against many diseases such as tuberculosis, irritations in mucous membranes and skin disorders. Silicon is found in apples, cherries, honey, grapes, asparagus, beets, onions, almonds, peanuts and the juices of the green leaves of most other vegetables. Deficiency can lead to soft brittle nails, ageing symptoms of skin such as wrinkles, thinning or loss of hair, poor bone development, insomnia and osteoporosis.

Fluorine

Fluorine is the element that prevents diseases from decaying the body. It is a germicide, and acts as an antidote to poison, sickness and disease. There is a strong affinity between calcium and fluorine. Fluorine is found in goat's milk, watercress, garlic, cauliflower, beets, cabbage, spinach and pistachio.

Minerals thus play an important role in every bodily function and are present in every human cell. Although the amount needed may be small, without even the trace of the mineral, dysfunction is bound to occur at some level in the body.

Benefits of Vegetarian Food

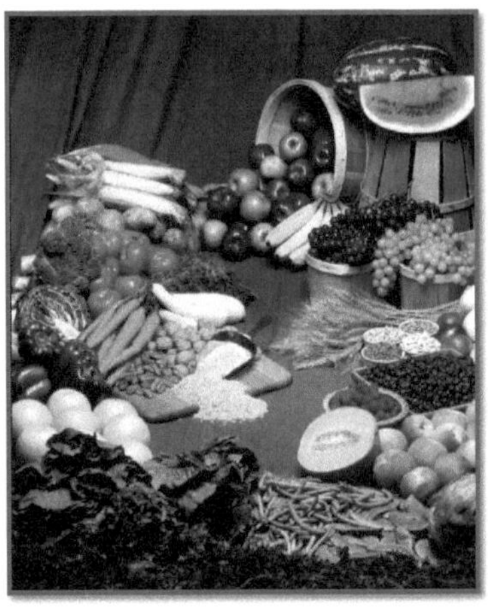

There are several significant benefits of vegetarian food in naturopathy. Protein in green vegetables is as high in quality as milk protein and thus makes a very valuable contribution to the vegetarian's protein nutrition. The high quality of protein balances the lower quality of other vegetarian proteins such as nuts and beans. A healthy and wholesome vegetarian diet can, as a result, easily meet the body's protein needs. A vegetarian diet can have a lot of nutritional benefits, if it is rich in fruits and vegetables, and contains moderate amounts of seeds, nuts, whole grains and legumes.

One of the most important benefits of a appropriate vegetarian diet is its low caloric content in relation to the bulk supplied, which helps maintain ideal weight. One more advantage of the vegetarian diet is the much lower intake of fat, if dairy products, seeds and nuts are eaten in moderation. This accounts for lower cholesterol levels found in vegetarians, which by far reduces the risk of developing heart diseases and breast and colon cancer. A third nutritional benefit of the vegetarian diet is its high fibre content. Fibre, being indigestible, increases the bulk of the faces, keeps them soft and makes them easy to expel.

One study has indicated that lacto-avo vegetarians consume twice as much and vagans four times as much fibre as non-vegetarians. High fibre intake has been related with decreased risks of diseases of the colon, appendicitis, cancer of the colon and rectum, hiatus hernia, piles and varicose veins. A perfectly constituted diet is one in which the principal ingredients are milk, milk products, any whole cereal grain or mixture of cereal grains, green leafy vegetables and fruits. These are the protective foods. They make well the defects of other constituents of the diet, guard the body against infection and disease of various kinds, and their use in adequate quantity ensures physical efficiency. Vegetarianism is thus a system based on scientific principles and has proved adequate for the best nutrition free from the poisons and bacteria of diseased animals. It is the best diet for man's best possible, physical, mental and spiritual development.

Importance of Dietary Fibre

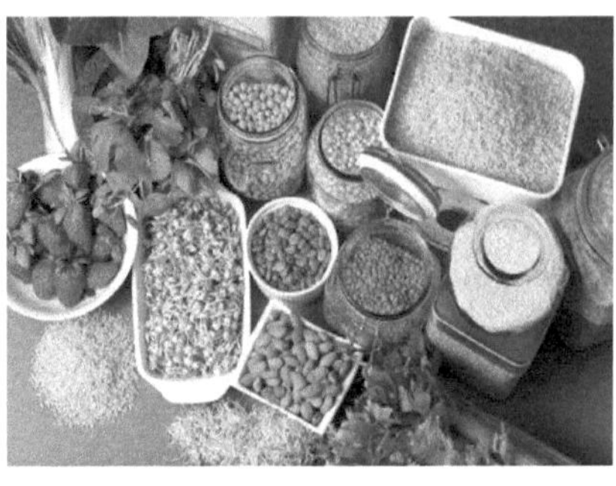

Importance of dietary fibres lies in the maintenance of health and prevention of diseases. Recent studies has shown the importance of dietary fibre and indicated that sufficient intake of fibre-rich diet may help avert obesity, colon cancer, heart disease, gallstones, irritable bowel syndrome, and diabetic conditions. Studies have also established that dietary fibre is a collection of elements with a variety of functions rather than a single substance with single function as was assumed earlier.

Fibre in the diet promotes more regular bowel movements and softer stools having increased weight. The softness of stools is basically due to the presence of emulsified gas which is produced by the bacterial action on the fibre. A high fibre intake results in better efficiency in the peristaltic movement of the colon. This helps in relieving the constipation which is the main cause of a number of acute and chronic diseases. Recent studies advocate that increasing the dietary fibre intake may be advantageous for patients with irritated bowel syndrome who have diarrhoea and rapid colonic transit, as well as to those who have constipation and slow transit. The high fibre diet, like bran, thus regulates the condition inside the colon so as to keep away from both extremes - constipation and Diarrhoea. Investigations have shown that several potential carcinogens are produced in the faeces.

Dietary fibre increases the bacteria in the large intestines which require nitrogen for their growth. This in turn diminishes the chances of cancerous changes in cells by reducing the amount of ammonia in the large bowel. Fibre reduces the absorption of cholesterol in the diet. It also slows down the rate of absorption of sugars from the food in the digestive system. Certain types of fibre boost the viscosity of the food content. This increased thickness indirectly reduces the need for insulin secreted by the pancreas. Thus a fibre-rich diet can help in diabetes mellitus. The most important food sources of fibre are unprocessed wheat bran, whole cereals, such as, rice, barley, Wheat, rye, millets; legumes such as beet, turnip, potato, carrots, and sweet potato; fruits like mango and guava and leafy vegetables such as cabbage, lettuce and celery.

The foods which are entirely devoid of fibre are fish, eggs, meat, milk, cheese, fats and sugars. Bran, the outer coverings of grains, is one of the richest sources of dietary fibre. Wheat and corn bran are extremely beneficial in relieving constipation. Experiments show that oat bran can reduce cholesterol levels to a great extent. Corn bran is considered more versatile. It relieves constipation and also lowers LDL cholesterol, which is one of the more harmful kinds. Besides being rich in fibre, bran has a real food value being rich in time, iron and vitamins and containing a considerable amount of protein. Legumes have high fibre content. Much of this fibre is water- soluble, which makes legumes likely agents for lowering cholesterol. Soyabeans, besides this, can also help control glucose levels. The types of fibre contained in vegetables and fruits contribute significantly towards good health. The vegetables with the biggest fibre ratings include potatoes, parsnips, sweet corn, carrots, and peas. Among the high ranking fruits are pears, raspberries, strawberries and guavas.

There are conflicting views as to the requirement of dietary fibre for good health. There is no recommended daily dietary allowance for it and hardly any data about optimum amounts. Excessive consumption of fibre, in particular bran, should however, be avoided. Due to its content of crude fibre, bran is comparatively harsh and it may irritate the delicate functioning of the digestive system, especially in the sick and the weak. Too much use of fibre may also result in loss of valuable minerals like calcium, phosphorus, magnesium and potassium from the body through excretion due to quick passage of food from the intestine.

Sprouts in Naturopathy

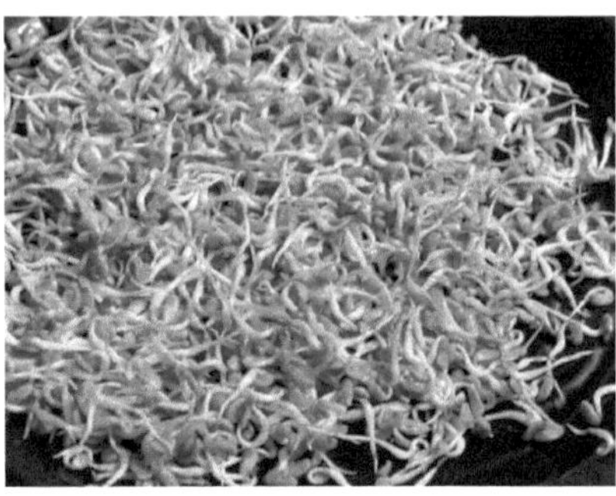

Sprouts in Naturopathy are regarded as the freshest and most nourishing of all vegetables in human diet. By a process of natural transmutation, sprouted food acquires immensely improved digestibility and nutritional qualities when compared to non sprouted embryo from which it derives. Sprouts supply all the necessary vitamins and minerals. They should form a very important component of the diet. Sprouting requires no constant care but only an occasional sprinkling of water. All edible grains, seeds and legumes can be sprouted.

Generally the following are used for sprouting:

- **Grains:** Wheat, bajra, maize, ragi and barley.
- **Seeds:** Alfalfa seeds, carrot seeds, coriander seeds, radish seeds, fenugreek seeds, pumpkin seeds and muskmelon seeds.
- **Legumes:** Mung, Bengal gram, groundnut and peas.

Alfalfa is the king of all sprouts. It is a vital component of human insulin. Apart from minerals, alfalfa is also a rich source of vitamins A, B, C, E and K and amino acids. Sesame seeds are another good source of nourishment. They include all the indispensable amino acids in their 20 per cent protein content and higher concentration of calcium than milk. They are high in lecithin, unsaturated fats, vitamin E and vitamin B complex, besides other live nutrients.

How to Sprout

As a first step, a high quality variety of seeds should be used for sprouting. It should be made sure that the seeds, legumes or grains are of the sproutable type. Soyabeans do not sprout well as they frequently become sour. It is wise to use seeds which are not chemically treated as this slows down the germination rate. The seeds should be washed carefully and then soaked overnight in a jar of pure water. The jar should be enclosed with cheesecloth or wire screening. The period of soaking will depend upon the size of the seed. Small seeds are soaked for five hours, medium size for eight hours and beans and grains for ten to twelve hours. On the next morning, the seeds should be rinsed and the water should be drained off. Not more than one fourth of the jar should be filled with the seeds for sprouting. Soaking makes the seeds, grains or legumes fatty, pulpy and full of water. It should, as a result, be ensured that the jar has enough room for the seeds to expand during sprouting. The seeds should be rinsed and water drained off three times every day till they are ready to eat. The seeds will germinate and become sprouts in two or three days from commencement of soaking, depending on temperature and humidity.

Benefits of Sprouts

There is a remarkable increase in nutrients in sprouted foods when compared to their dried embryo. In the process of sprouting, the vitamins, minerals and protein increase significantly with corresponding reduce in calories and carbohydrate content. These comparisons are based on equivalent water content in the foods measured. Analysis of dried seeds, grains and legumes shows a very low water content. But this increases up to tenfold when the same food is converted into sprouts. For precise comparison each must be brought to a common denomination of equal water content to assess the exact change brought in nutritional value. The increase in protein accessibility is of great importance. It is a valuable indicator of the enhanced nutritional value of a food when sprouted.

The remarkable increase in sodium content supports the analysis that sprouted foods offer nutritional qualities. Sodium is vital to the digestive process within the gastro-intestinal tract and also to the elimination of carbon dioxide. Dried seeds, grains and legumes do not contain noticeable traces of ascorbic acid, yet when sprouted, they divulge quite important quantities which are significant in the body's capacity to metabolise proteins. The countless increase in ascorbic acid derives from their absorption of atmospheric elements at the time of growth. Sprouts have quite a lot of other benefits. They contribute food in predigested form, that is, the food which has already been acted upon by the enzymes and made to digest without difficulty.

Sprouts are an enormously inexpensive method of obtaining a concentration of vitamins, minerals and enzymes. They have in them all the component nutrients of fruits and vegetables and are `live` foods. Eating sprouts is the safest and best way of getting the advantage of both fruits and vegetables without contamination and harmful insecticides. It should, however, be ensured that seeds and dried beans are purchased from a store where they are fresh, unsprayed and packaged as food. Seeds that are packaged for planting purposes may contain mercury compounds or other toxic chemicals.

Naturopathy and Diseases

Naturopathy, though, is considered to be of a very recent origin but it involves ancient methods of nature cure for several diseases. Naturopathy is a constructive method of treatment which aims at removing the basic cause of disease through the rational use of the elements freely available in nature. It was practiced in ancient Egypt, Greece and Rome. Hippocrates, the father of medicine, strongly advocated it. There are references in India's ancient sacred books about the widespread use of nature's excellent healing agents such as air, earth, water and sun. It is not only a system of healing, but also a way of life, in tune with the internal vital forces or natural elements comprising the human body. It is a complete revolution in the art and science of living.

Naturopathy is based on the realisation that man is born healthy and strong and that he can stay as such as living in accord with the laws of nature. Even if born with some inherited affliction, the individual can get rid of it by putting to the best use the natural agents of healing. Fresh air, sunshine, a proper diet, exercise, scientific relaxation, constructive thinking and the right mental attitude, along with prayer and meditation all play their part in keeping a sound mind in a sound body. Nature cure believes that disease is an unusual condition of the body resulting from the defiance of the natural laws. Every such violation has repercussions on the human system in the shape of lowered vitality, irregularities of the blood and lymph and the accumulation of waste matter and toxins. Thus, through a faulty diet it is not the digestive system alone which is adversely affected. When toxins accumulate, other organs such as the bowels, kidneys, skin and lungs are overworked and cannot get rid of these harmful substances as quickly as they are produced. Besides this, mental and emotional disturbances cause imbalances of the vital electric field within which cell metabolism takes place, producing toxins.

The first and most basic principle of naturopathy is that all forms of disease are due to the same cause, namely, the accumulations of waste materials and bodily refuse in the system. These waste materials in the healthy individual are detached from the system through the organs of elimination. But in the diseased person, they are steadily piling up in the body through years of defective habits of living such as wrong feeding, improper care of the body and habits contributing to enervation and nervous exhaustion such as worry, overwork and excesses of all kinds. It follows from this basic principle that the only way to cure disease is to employ methods which will enable the system to throw off these toxic accumulations. The second basic principle of nature cure is that all acute diseases such as fever, colds, inflammations, digestive disturbances and skin eruptions are nothing more than self-initiated efforts on the part of the body to throw off the accumulated waste materials and that all chronic diseases such as heart disease, diabetes, rheumatism, asthma, kidney disorders, are the results of continued suppression of the acute diseases through harmful methods such as drugs, vaccines, narcotics and gland extracts. The third principle of nature cure is that the body contains an elaborate healing mechanism which has the power to bring about a return to normal condition of health, provided right methods are employed to enable it to do so. In other words, the power to cure disease lies within the body itself and not in the hands of the doctor.

To cure disease in Naturopathy, the first and foremost requirement is to regulate the diet. To get rid of accumulated toxins and restore the equilibrium of the system, it is desirable to completely exclude acid forming foods, including proteins, starches and fats, for a week or more and to confine the diet to fresh fruits which will disinfect the stomach and alimentary canal. If the body is overloaded with morbid matter, as in acute disease, a complete fast for a few days may be necessary for the elimination of toxins. Fruit juice may, however, be taken during a fast. Alkaline foods such as raw vegetables and sprouted whole grain cereals may be added after a week of a fruits-only diet.

In general, naturopathy investigates scientifically all the methods and procedures which are related to the improvement of ills and the maintenance of sound health. Naturopathy prohibits the use of poisonous drugs, serums, invasive surgery, x-ray and radiation for remedial purposes.

Chapter 1

Acne

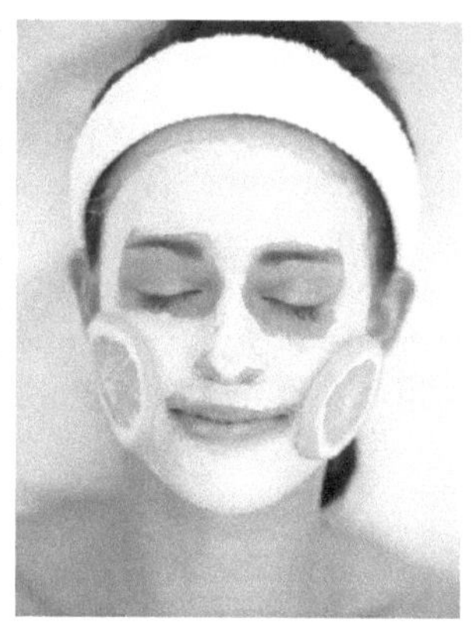

Natural cure for acne in naturopathy importance is given on the diet and water applications. The patient is recommended to resort to all fruit diet for about a week. In this routine, there should be three meals a day, consisting of fresh juicy fruits, such as apples, pears, grapes, grape-fruit, pineapple and peaches. Citrus fruits such as bananas, dried, stewed or tinned fruits should not be taken. Unsweetened lemon or plain water, either hot or cold, should be drunk and nothing else. During this period, warm water enema should be taken daily to cleanse the bowels and all other measures adopted to eliminate constipation.

After a week of all fruit diet, the patient can gradually adopt a well-balanced diet. Emphasis should be on raw foods, mainly fresh fruits and vegetables, sprouted seeds, raw nuts and whole grain cereals, especially millet and brown rice. Further shorter periods on the all-fruits for three days, or so may be necessary at a monthly interval till the condition of the skin improves. Strict attention to diet is essential for improvement. Starchy, protein and fatty foods should be avoided. Meats, sugar, strong tea or coffee, condiments, pickles, refined and processed foods should all be avoided, as also soft drinks, candies, ice cream and products made with sugar and white flour. Two vitamins, namely, niacin and vitamin A have been used successfully to treat acne. Another effective remedy in the area of nutrition that seems to offer new promise of help for acne is zinc. It has shown dramatic results in some cases.

As regards local treatment in case of acne, hot fomentation should be applied to open up the pores and squeeze the waste matter. Then it should be rinsed with cold water. Sun and air baths by exposing the whole body to sun and air are highly beneficial. The healing packs made of grated cucumber, oatmeal cooked in milk, and cooked, creamed carrots used externally, have been found to be effective. The orange peel is valuable in the treatment of acne. The peel, pounded well with water on a piece of stone, should be applied to the affected areas. The lemon has also proved useful in removing pimples and acne. It should be applied on a regular basis. A teaspoonful of coriander juice, mixed with a pinch of turmeric powder, is another effective home remedy for pimples and blackheads. The mixture should be applied to the face after thoroughly washing it, every night before retiring.

The juice of raw potatoes has also proved very valuable in clearing skin blemishes. This cleansing results from high content of potassium sulphur, phosphorous and chlorine in the potato. These elements are, however, of value only when the potato is raw as in this state they are composed of live organic atoms. A hot Epsom-salt bath twice a week will be highly beneficial in all cases of acne.

Chapter 2

Cataract

Natural remedy for cataract in naturopathy is possible if it is detected at an early stage. A thorough course of cleansing the system of the toxic matter is necessary. It is beneficial to go through a fast for three to four days on orange juice and water. Warm water enema may be taken during this period. After this initial fast, a diet of very controlled nature should be followed for two weeks. In this regimen, breakfast may consist of oranges or grapes or any other juicy fruit in season. Raw vegetable salads in season, with olive oil and lemon juice dressing, and soaked raisins, figs or dates should be taken during lunch. Evening meals may comprise vegetable such as spinach, fenugreek, drum sticks, cabbage, cauliflower, and carrot, turnips, steamed in their own juices, and a few nuts or some fruits, such as apples, pears and grapes. No bread or any other food should be added to this diet.

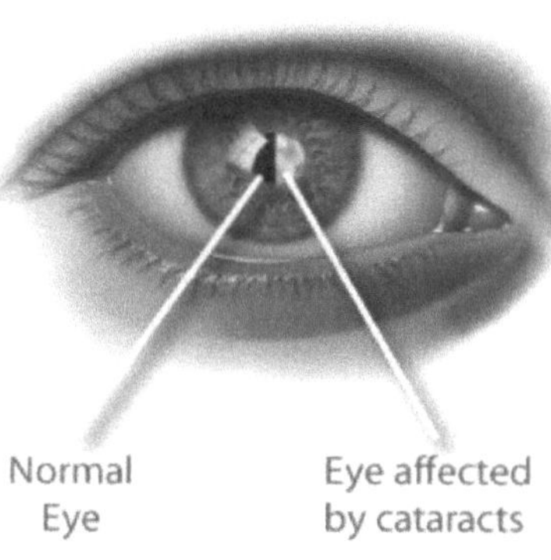

After two weeks on this diet, the cataract patient may start on a fuller diet on the following lines:

- **Breakfast:** Any fresh fruits in season, except bananas.
- **Lunch:** A large mixed raw vegetable salad with whole meal bread or chapatis and butter.
- **Dinner:** Two or three steamed vegetables, other than potatoes, with nuts and fresh fruit.

The short fast followed by a restricted diet should be repeated after three months of the commencement of the treatment and again three months later, if required. The bowels should be cleansed daily with a warm water enema during the fast, and afterwards as necessary. The patient should avoid white bread, sugar, refined cereals, rice, boiled potatoes, puddings and pies, strong tea or coffee, alcoholic beverages, condiments, pickles, sauces or other so-called aids to digestion.

There is increasing evidence to show that in several cases cataracts have actually been upturned by appropriate nutritional treatment. However, the time needed for such cure may extend from six months to three years. The aniseed is considered a valuable remedy for cataract. The patient should take about six grams of aniseed daily in the morning and evening. Equal weights of aniseed and coriander powder and mixed with brown sugar is also beneficial in the treatment of this disease and the mixture should be taken in doses of twelve grams in the morning and evening. Another helpful remedy for cataract is to grind seven kernels of almonds and half a gram of pepper together in water, and then drink the mixture after sifting and sweetening the mixture with sugar candy. It helps the eyes to recover their vigour. Simultaneous with the dietary treatment, the patient should adopt various methods of relaxing and strengthening the eyes. These include moving the eyes gently up and down, from side to side and in a circle, clock-wise and anti-clockwise; rotating the neck in circles and semi-circles and briskly moving the shoulders clock-wise and anti-clockwise.

The patient should also resort to palming which is highly beneficial in removing strain and relaxing the eyes and its surrounding tissues. The Epsom salt bath is highly beneficial and should be taken twice a week. The patient should remain in the bath from twenty five to thirty five minutes till he perspires freely. After the bath the patient should cool off gradually. Closed eyes should also be bathed at least twice daily with hot water containing Epsom salt - a tablespoonful of salt to a large cupful of hot water. In cases where the cataract has been caused by stress, an anti stress diet rich in protein, vitamin B,C, E, pantothenic acid and nutrients is indispensable to overcome the trouble. If a cataract has already developed, the diet will help prevent its occurrence in the other type. Fresh air and gentle outdoor exercises, such as walking, are other essentials to the treatment. Exposure to heat and bright light should be avoided as far as possible.

Chapter 3

Common Cold

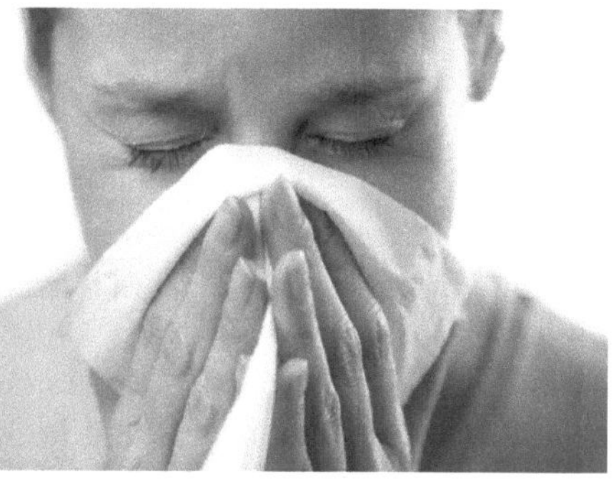

Natural remedy for common cold prescribes for a proper diet. The treatment should begin with by putting the patient on a fast for two days. Nothing should be taken during this period except warm water mixed with lemon juice and honey or fruit juice and hot water. A liquid diet of fruit juice in large amounts is essential to neutralise the acid condition of the blood and hot drinks are required to help clear the kidneys. Pineapple juice in particular is highly advantageous. A warm water enema should be used on a daily basis to cleanse the bowels during this period.

The short juice fast may be followed by an exclusive fresh fruit diet for three days. In this regimen, the patient should have three meals a day of fresh fruits such as apples, pears, grapes, oranges, pineapple, peaches, melon or any other juicy fruits in season. Bananas, dried or stewed or tinned fruits, should not be taken. After the fruit diet, the patient should gradually intake a well-balanced diet of three basic food groups, namely (i) seeds, nuts and grains (ii) vegetables and (iii) fruits. It is advisable to avoid meat, fish, eggs, cheese and starchy foods for a few days. The patient should toughen the system as a whole by taking a diet which supplies all the vitamins and minerals the body needs. Vitamin C protects one against infection and acts as harmless antibiotics. It is found in citrus fruits, green leafy vegetables, sprouted Bengal and green grams. Lime is the most vital among the many home remedies for common cold. It should be taken well diluted. Lime juice should be diluted in a glass of warm water, and a teaspoonful of honey should be added to it. It forms an ideal remedy for a cold and dry cough.

Garlic soup is a very old medication to reduce the severity of cold. Garlic contains antiseptic and antispasmodic properties besides a number of other medicinal virtues. The volatile oil in garlic flushes out the system of all toxins and thus helps bring down fever. Garlic oil combined with onion juice, diluted with water and drunk several times a day, has also been found in several studies to be enormously effective in the cure of the common cold. Ginger is also an excellent food remedy for colds and coughs. Ginger should be cut into small pieces and boiled in a cup of water; it should then be strained and half a teaspoon of sugar added to it. Ginger tea, prepared by adding a few pieces of ginger into boiled water before adding tea leaves, is also an effective remedy for colds and for fevers resulting from cold.

Turmeric, with its antiseptic properties, is an effective remedy for cold and throat irritations. Half a teaspoonful of fresh turmeric powder mixed in thirty grams of warm milk is a useful prescription for these conditions. Turmeric powder should be put into a hot ladle. Milk should then be poured in it and boiled over a slow fire. In case of a running cold, smoke from the burning turmeric should be inhaled. It will increase the discharge from the nose and will bring faster relief.

A hot water bath, is recommended as it helps relieve much of the congestion in the chest and nasal membranes. Hot packs or fomentations are excellent for treating chest and head colds. Steam bath, hot foot bath and hot hip bath are also useful as they kindle perspiration. Steam inhalation will help alleviate the congestion of the nasal tissues. Gargling with hot water mixed with salt is beneficial for a sore throat. Cold chest packs should be applied two or three times a day as they will relieve congestion of lungs and help in eliminating the accumulated mucus. Other useful measures in the treatment of common cold are mild sunbath, fresh air and deep breathing, brisk walks, sound sleep, adjustment of one's clothes and habits to the requirements of the season, so as to invalidate the effect of weather fluctuations. Yogasanas like bhujangasana, salabhasana, dhanurasana, and yogamudra in vajrasana, yogic kriyas such as jalneti and vamandhouti and pranayamas such as kapalbhati, anuloma- viloma and suryabhedana are beneficial in the treatment of the common cold.

Chapter 4

Anaemia

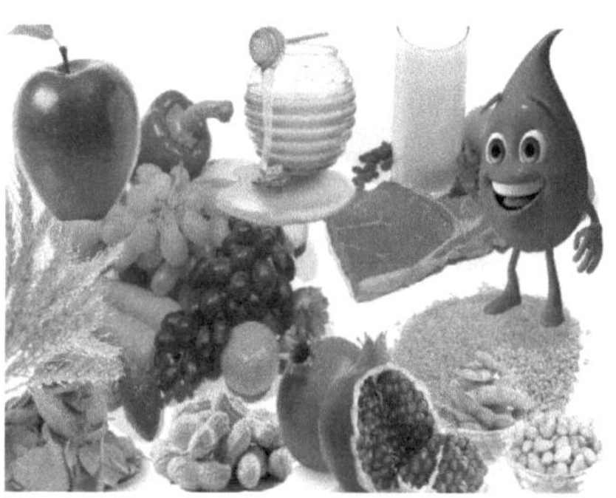

In the natural cure of anaemia, diet is of supreme significance. Almost every nutrient is needed for the production of red blood cells, haemoglobin and the enzymes, required for their synthesis. Refined food like white bread, polished rice, sugar, and desserts prepare the body for the much required iron. Iron should always be taken in its natural organic form as the use of inorganic can prove harmful, destroying the protective vitamins and unsaturated fatty acids, causing serious liver damage and even miscarriage and delayed or premature births. The common foods rich in natural organic iron are wheat and wheat grain cereals, brown rice, green leafy vegetables, cabbage, carrot, celery, beets, tomatoes, spinach ; fruits like apples, berries, cherries, grapes, raisins, figs, dates, peaches and eggs. It has been proved that a generous intake of iron alone will not help in the regeneration of haemoglobin. The supplies of protein, too, should be adequate. The diet should, therefore, be adequate in proteins of high biological value such as those found in milk, cheese and egg.

Copper is also vital for the utilisation of iron in the building of haemoglobin. Vitamin B12 is a must for preventing or curing anaemia. This vitamin is usually found in animal protein and especially in organic meats like kidney and liver. A heavy meat diet is often associated with a high haemoglobin and high red cell count, but it has its disadvantages. One cause of anaemia is intestinal putrefaction, which is primarily brought on by a high meat diet. There are, however, other equally good alternative sources of vitamin B12 such as dairy products, like milk, eggs and cheese, peanuts. Wheat germ and soyabeans also contain some B12. Vegetarians should include sizeable amounts of milk, milk products and eggs in their diet. For prevention of anaemia, it is essential to take the entire B-complex range which includes B_{12}, as well as the natural foods mentioned above.

A liberal intake of ascorbic acid is necessary to facilitate absorption of iron. At least two helpings of citrus fruits and other ascorbic acid rich foods should be taken daily. Mention must be made of beets which are extremely important in curing anaemia. Beet juice contains potassium, phosphorous, calcium, sulphur, iodine, iron, copper, carbohydrates, protein, and fat, vitamins, B1, B_2, niacin B_6, C and vitamin P. With its high iron content, beet juice regenerates and reactivates the red blood cells, supplies the body with fresh oxygen and helps the normal function of vesicular breathing.

Water treatment is also an important part of Indian naturopathy. A cold water bath is among the most valuable curative measures in anaemia. The patient should be given carefully graduated cold baths twice daily. Hot Epsom salt bath for five to ten minutes once a week and an occasional cabinet steam bath are also recommended. Full sun baths are especially beneficial as sunlight stimulates the production of red cells. There are other important factors which are helpful in curing anaemia. Deep breathing and light exercise like walking and simple yoga asanas should be undertaken to tone up the system. Massage therapy also helps to keep the blood level high.

Chapter 5

Arthritis

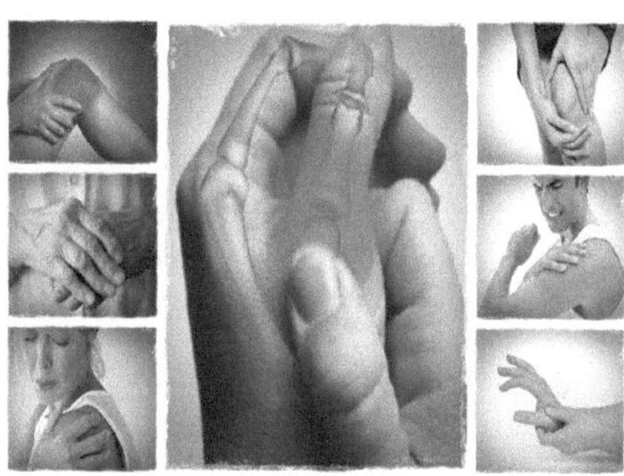

Diet is of supreme importance for the natural cure of arthritis. Diet therapy of the arthritis patient should be planned along alkaline lines and should include fruits and vegetables for protection and proteins and carbohydrates for energy. It may consist of a couple of fresh raw vegetables in the form of a salad and at least two cooked vegetables. Cabbage, carrot, cucumber, endive, lettuce, onion, tomatoes and watercress may be used for a raw salad. The cooked vegetables may consist of asparagus, beets, cauliflower, cabbage, carrots, celery, mushroom, onions, peas, spinach, tomatoes, squash and turnips.

In severe cases of arthritis, it is wise to put the patient on raw vegetables juice therapy for about a week. Green juice, extracted from any green leafy vegetable, mixed with carrot, celery and red beet juice, is precise for arthritis. The alkaline action of raw juices dissolves the accumulation of deposits around the joints and in other tissues. Fresh pineapple is also valuable as the enzyme in fresh pineapple juice, reduces swelling and inflammation in osteoarthritis and rheumatoid arthritis. Repeated juice fasts are recommended at intervals of every two months. The raw potato juice therapy is regarded one of the most successful biological treatments for rheumatic and arthritic conditions.

Black gingerly seeds, soaked overnight in water, have been found to be helpful in preventing everyday joint pains. The water in which the seeds are soaked should also be taken along with the seeds the first thing in the morning. Drinking water kept overnight in a copper container also serves the same purpose. This water has traces of copper which helps strengthen the muscular system. For the same reason wearing a copper ring or bracelet will also help. Warm coconut oil or mustard oil, mixed with camphor should be massaged in case of stiff and aching joints. It will enhance blood supply and reduce inflammation and stiffness on account of gentle warmth produced while massaging. Camphorated oil is used for the purpose.

Other remedies found useful in relieving pains in the joints comprise green gram soup mixed with crushed garlic cloves and a teaspoonful of powdered fenugreek seeds in warm water taken daily. Sea bathing is considered beneficial in the treatment of arthritis. The natural iodine in the sea water is said to relieve arthritis pain. If sea bathing is not possible, the patient should relax for thirty minutes every night in a tub of warm water in which a cupful of sea salt has been mixed. The minerals in the sea salt, especially iodine, can be absorbed through the skin pores. Rest is of greatest importance to arthritis, and patients should not overdo their work, exercise or recreation activities.

Constipation should be avoided as it poisons the system and adds to the irritation and inflammation of the joints. Light exercises such as walking, hiking and swimming are advantageous. Maintaining a normal body weight is also a vital factor in preventing arthritis. The yoga asanas helpful in curing arthritis are trikonasana, bhujangasana, salabhasana, naukasana, vakrasana and shavasana. Arthritis patients should practice these asanas regularly. Neutral immersion baths, hot foot baths, ultrasonic diathermy and exposure of the affected parts to infra-red rays, a knee pack applied for an hour every night, stream baths and a massage once a week are beneficial in the treatment of arthritis. All general cold water treatments, such as cold baths and cold sprays, should be avoided.

Chapter 6

Conjunctivitis

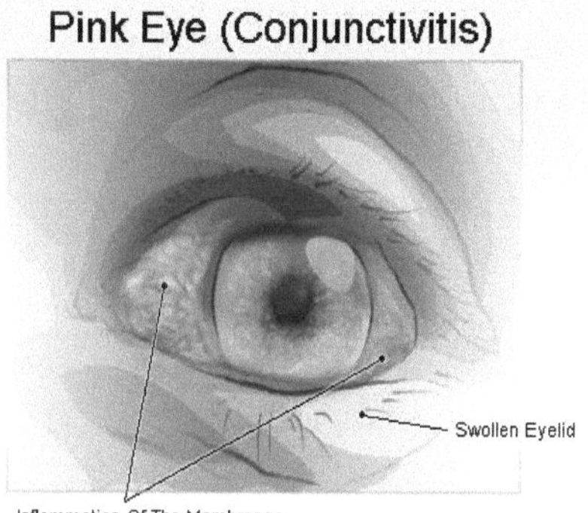

Natural remedy for Conjunctivitis begins with an exclusive fresh fruit diet for about seven days. The diet may include fresh juicy fruits in season such as apple, orange, pears, grapes, pineapple and grapefruit. Those who have a serious trouble should undertake a juice fast for three or four days. The method is to take the juice of an orange, in a glass of warm water, if desired, every two hours from 8 a.m. to 8 p.m. Nothing else should be taken as otherwise the value of the fast will be lost. If orange juice disagrees, carrot juice may be taken. A warm water enema should be taken on a daily basis during the period of fasting.

The short juice fast may be followed by an all-fruit diet for further seven days. **Thereafter, the patient may adopt a general diet scheme on the following lines:**

- **Breakfast:** Any fresh fruits in season, except bananas.
- **Lunch:** Large mixed raw vegetable salad with whole meat bread or chapatis and butter.
- **Dinner:** Two or three steamed vegetables, other than potatoes, with nuts and fresh fruit.

The patient should avoid too much intake of starchy and sugary foods in the form of white bread, refined cereals, potatoes, puddings, pies, pastry, sugar, jams and confectionery, which cause the general catarrhal condition as well as conjunctivitis. He should also avoid the eating of excessive quantities of meat and other protein and fatty foods, strong tea and coffee, too much salt, condiments and sauces.

Raw juices of certain vegetables, especially carrots, and spinach, have been found helpful in the treatment of conjunctivitis. The combined juices of these two vegetables have proved very effectual. 200 ml. of spinach juice should be mixed with 300 ml. of carrot juice in this combination. Vitamin A and B2 have also been found valuable in the treatment of conjunctivitis. The patient should take moderate quantities of natural foods rich in these two vitamins. Valuable sources of vitamin A are: whole milk, curds, butter, carrots, pumpkin, green leafy vegetables, tomatoes, mangoes and papaya. Foods rich in vitamin B2 are green leafy vegetables, milk, almonds, citrus fruits, bananas and tomatoes.

As regards local treatment, a cold foment renders almost immediate relief by chasing away an overactive local blood supply. First a small hand towel should be folded and saturated with cold water. The excess water should be squeezed out and the towel should be applied gently over both eyes. It should be covered with a piece of warm cloth to retain the temperature. It is advisable to carry out the procedure for one hour. After terminating the wet pack treatment, the eyes are to be covered with a dry towel. The damaged eye tissues will quickly return to normal. The treatment should be repeated every night for a week, even though the problem may clear up with the first treatment itself. The eye muscle exercises on defective vision are also valuable in the treatment of conjunctivitis.

Chapter 7

Depression

Naturopathy offers a natural remedy to depression. Diet has a profound effect on the mental health of a person. Even a single nutritional deficiency can cause depression in susceptible people. Activity and exercise also have a profound effect on the mental state of a person. Relaxation enables the muscles to work more efficiently and eliminates fatigue by promoting venous blood circulation throughout the body. Thus in naturopathy the treatment of depression consists of regulating the diet, exercise, scientific relaxation and meditation.

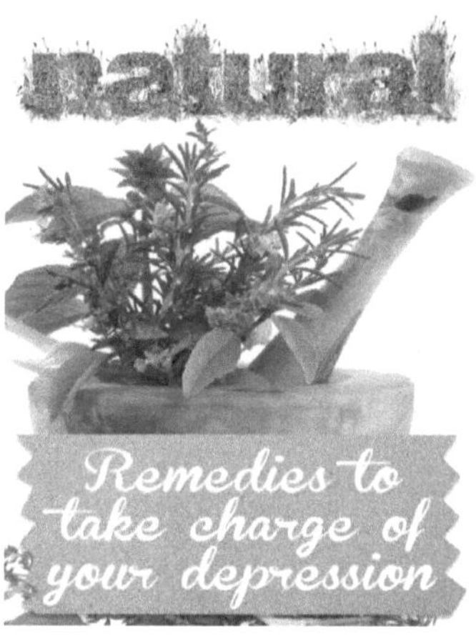

The diet of persons suffering from depression should entirely exclude tea, coffee, alcohol, chocolate and cola, all white flour products, sugar, chemical additives, white rice and strong condiments. The diet should be restricted to three meals. Fruits can be taken in the morning for breakfast with milk and a handful of nuts and seeds. Lunch may comprise steamed vegetables, whole wheat chappatis and a glass of butter-milk. For dinner, green vegetable salad and all accessible sprouts such as alfalfa seeds, cottage cheese or a glass of butter-milk would be best.

The depressive mood can be defeated by activity. Those who are depressive will forget their misery by doing something. At home they can take to decorating, repairing or constructing something new. The pleasure of achievement overcomes the anguish of misery. Exercise also plays an important role in the treatment of depression. It not only keeps the body physically and mentally fit but also provides amusement and mental relaxation. Exercise produces chemical and psychological changes that improve mental health. Exercise may also recover the function of the autonomic nervous system. Exercise also gives a feeling of accomplishment and thus reduces the sense of vulnerability. Some form of active exercise, must be undertaken each day at a regular hour. Walking is one such exercise.

Yogic asanas such as vakrasana, bhujangasana, salabhasana, halasana, paschimottanasana, sarvangasana and shavasana and pranayamas like kapalbhati, anuloma-viloma and bhastrika are highly advantageous in the treatment of depression.

The patient must gain control over his nervous system and channelise his mental and emotional activities into relaxing harmonious vibrations. This can be achieved by ensuring sufficient rest and sleep under right conditions. The best method of relaxation is to practice shavasana. Meditation involves training the mind to remain fixed on a certain external or internal location. Meditation will help create an amount of balance in the nervous system. Regularity of time, place and practice are very vital in meditation. Regularity conditions the mind to slowing down its activities with a minimum delay.

A neutral immersion bath for one hour daily is also useful in the treatment of depression. This bath is administered in a bath tub which should be appropriately fitted with hot and cold water connections. The patient should lie in the tub after filling it with water at a temperature ranging from 92 degrees to 98 degrees Fahrenheit. The head should be kept cold with a cold compress.

Chapter 7

Dysentery

Natural remedy for dysentery involves a fasting therapy and should aim at the removal of the toxins from the system. The patient should fast as long as acute symptoms are present. During the period of fasting, only orange juice and water should be taken. In the alternative, the patient should subsist on buttermilk till the acute symptoms are over. Butter milk battles offending bacteria and helps establishment of helpful micro-organisms in the intestines. The patient may be given small doses of castor oil in the form of mixture. In addition to administration of castor oil, the mechanical exclusion of accumulated poisonous matter should be attempted by giving very low pressure enema, admitting as much water as the patient can tolerate.

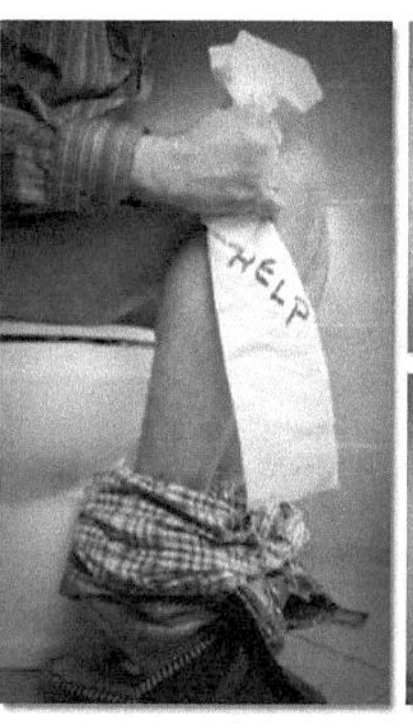

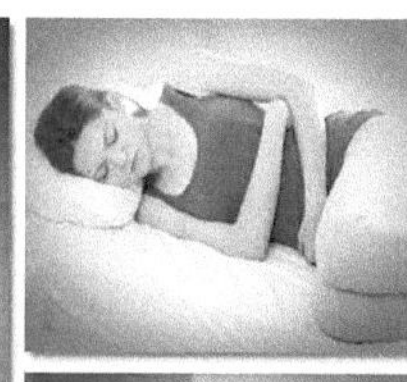

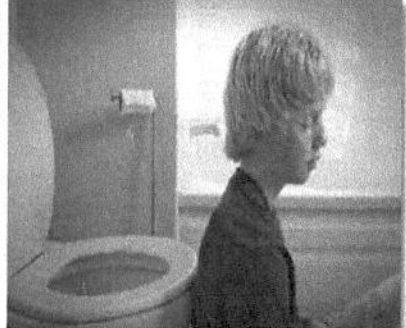

Complete bed rest is advisable as movement induces pain and aggravates distressing symptoms. A hot water bag may be applied over the abdomen. After the acute symptoms are over, the patient may be allowed rice, curd, fresh ripe fruits, especially bael, banana and pomegranate and skimmed milk. Solid foods should be introduced very cautiously and gradually according to the pace of recuperation. Flesh foods of all kinds should be avoided in future as far as possible. Other foods which should be avoided are tea, coffee, white sugar and white flour and products made from them as well as alcohol in all forms. Foods which have a detoxifying and cleansing effect upon the intestines on their passage, through, such as fruits and vegetables, are most vital to a future dietary.

Among specific food remedies, bael fruit is, perhaps, the most effective in the healing of dysentery of both the varieties. Pulp of the fruit mixed with jaggery should be given thrice daily. To deal with a chronic case of dysentery, unripe bael fruit is roasted over the fire and the pulp is mixed with water. Large quantities of the mixture so made should be administered with jaggery. The pulp of the unripe fruit mixed with an equal quantity of dried ginger can also be given with butter milk. The use of pomegranate rind is another effective therapy for dysentery. Lemon juice is very effective in dealing with ordinary cases of dysentery. Other remedies considered useful in the treatment of dysentery are the use of small pieces of onions mixed with curd and equal parts of the tender leaves of the peepal tree, coriander leaves and sugar chewed slowly.

Chapter 8

Gall Bladder Stones

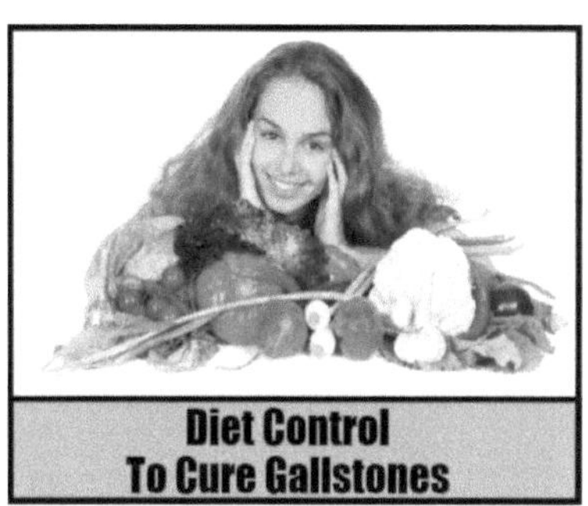
Diet Control
To Cure Gallstones

Natural remedy for gall bladder stone is possible in case of smaller gall stones. Diet is the fundamental part in the treatment of gall bladder disorders. In cases of acute gall-bladder inflammation, the patient should fast for two or three days, until the acute condition clears. Nothing but water should be taken during the fast. After the fast, the patient should take carrot, beet, grape fruit, lemon and grape juice for a few days. The diet should contain a sufficient amount of lacto-vegetarian, consisting of raw and cooked vegetables, vegetable juices, and a moderate amount of fruit and seeds. Yogurt, cottage cheese and a tablespoon of olive oil twice a day should also be taken.

All meats, eggs, animal fats and processed and denatured fats as well as fried foods should be avoided. The diet should also keep out refined carbohydrates, particularly sugar, sugar products, alcohol, soft drinks, cakes, puddings, ice-cream, coffee and citrus fruits. The patient should eat small meals at regular intervals, rather than three large meals.

The following is the suggested menu for those suffering from gall-bladder disorders:

- **Breakfast:** Fresh fruit, one or two slices of whole meal toast and a cup of skimmed powder milk.
- **Mid morning:** Fresh fruit juice.
- **Lunch:** Vegetable soup, a large salad consisting of vegetables in season with dressing of lemon or vegetable oil.
- **Dinner:** Vegetable oil, one or two lightly cooked vegetables, baked potato, brown rice or whole wheat chappati and a glass of buttermilk.

Regular applications of hot and cold fomentations to the abdomen improve the circulation of the liver and gall-bladder. They also stimulate concentrations of the gall-bladder, thereby improving the flow of bile. A cold hip bath improves the general abdominal tone. The pain of gall-stone colic can be relieved by the application of hot packs or fomentation to the upper abdominal area. A warm water enema at body temperature will help eliminate faecal accumulations if the patient is constipated. Exercise is necessary as physical inactivity can lead to lazy gall-bladder type indigestion which may eventually result in the formation of stones. Yogic asanas which are beneficial in toning up the liver and gall-bladder are: sarvangasana, paschimottanasana, salabhasana, dhanurasana and bhujangasana.

Chapter 9

Glaucoma

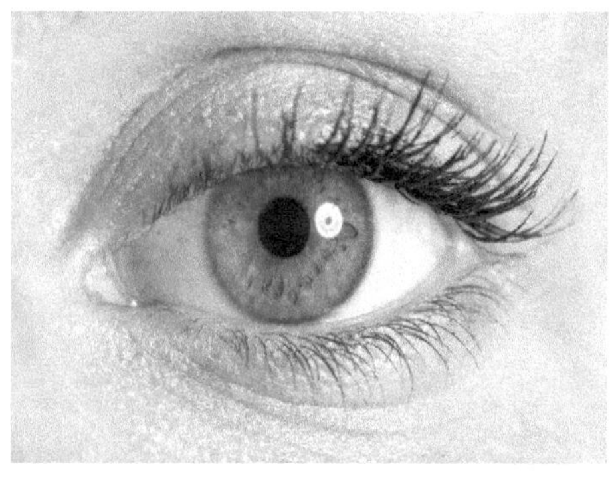

Natural treatment for glaucoma is same as that for any other condition associated with high toxicity and is directed towards preserving whatever sight remains. Though cases of advanced glaucoma may be beyond a cure, even so certain nutritional and other biological approaches can prove effective in controlling the condition and preserving the remaining sight. If treated in the early stages, the results are encouraging. Diet is an important factor in the treatment of Glaucoma. Certain foodstuff should be meticulously avoided by patients afflicted from glaucoma. Coffee in particular, should be totally avoided because of its high caffeine content. Beer and tobacco, which can cause constriction of blood vessels, should also be avoided. Tea should be taken only in moderate quantity. The patient should not take excessive fluids, whether it is juice, milk or water at any time. He may drink small amounts a number of times with at least one hour intervals.

The diet of the patient suffering from glaucoma should be based on three basic food groups, namely, seeds, nuts and grains; vegetables and fruit, with emphasis on raw vitamin C-rich foods, fresh fruits and vegetables. The breakfast may consist of oranges or grapes or any other juicy fruits in season and a handful of raw nuts or seeds. A raw vegetable salad with olive oil and lemon juice dressing, two or three whole wheat chappatis and a glass of buttermilk may be taken for lunch. The dinner may comprise steamed vegetables, butter and cottage cheese.

Certain nutrients have been found helpful in the treatment of glaucoma. It has been found that the glaucoma patients are generally deficient in vitamins A, B, C, protein, calcium and other minerals. Nutrients such as calcium and B complex have proved advantageous in relieving the intraocular condition. Many practitioners believe that intraocular pressure in glaucoma can be lowered by vitamin C therapy. The patient should embark on various methods of relaxing and strengthening the eyes. He should keep away from emotional stress and develop a peaceful, restful life style. He should also avoid prolonged straining of the eyes such as occurs during excessive television or movie watching and too much reading. The use of sun glasses should be avoided.

Chapter 10

High Blood Pressure

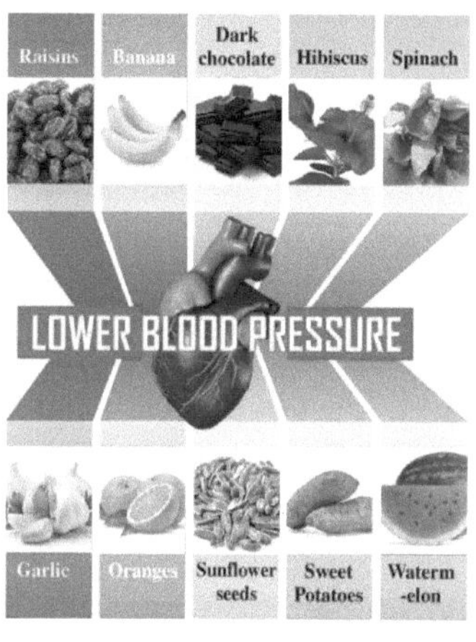

Natural cure for high blood pressure is to follow a well-balanced routine of proper diet, exercise and rest. Diet is the most important part of the treatment. Meat and eggs cause the blood pressure to rise more than any other food. The pressure is lowered and blood clotting is diminished by consuming a higher fruit content, lower protein and non-flesh diet. A natural diet comprises fresh fruits and vegetables. A hypertension patient should start the process of medication by living on an exclusive fruit-diet for at least a week, and take fruits at five-hourly intervals thrice in the day. Oranges, apples, pears, mangoes, guava, raspberry, and water-melon are the best diet in such cases. Milk may be taken after a week of `fruits only` diet. The milk should be fresh and should be boiled only once. The patient can be permitted cereals in his food after two weeks.

Vegetables if taken raw are helpful for the patients of hypertension. If they are cooked, it should be ensured that their natural juices are not burnt in the process of cooking. Vegetables like cucumber, carrot, tomatoes, onion, cabbage and spinach are best taken in their raw form. They may be cut into small pieces and sprinkled with a little salt and the juice of a lemon added to them so as to make them more appetising. Garlic is regarded as one of the most effectual remedies to lower blood pressure. The pressure and tension are reduced because it has the power to ease the spasms of the small arteries. Garlic also slows the pulse and modifies the heart rhythm besides relieving the symptoms of dizziness, numbness, and shortness of breath and the formation of gas within the digestive tract.

Another effective food remedy for high blood pressure is Indian gooseberry (amla). A tablespoonful each of fresh amla juice and honey mixed together should be taken every morning in this condition. Lemon is also regarded as an important food to control high blood pressure. It is a rich source of vitamin P which is found both in the juice and peel of the fruit. This vitamin is necessary for preventing capillary fragility. Watermelon is another valuable protection against high blood pressure. Recent studies have revealed an important link between dietary calcium and potassium and hypertension. Researchers have found that people who take potassium rich diets have a low incidence of hypertension even if they do not control their salt intake. They have also found that people with hypertension do not seem to get much calcium in the form of dairy products.

Exercise plays an indispensable part of curing hypertension. Walking is an excellent form of exercise. It helps to relieve tension, builds up the muscles and aids in the circulation of blood. As the blood pressure shows signs of lessening, more exercise like bicycling, swimming, jogging should be taken. Yoga asanas such as surya namaskar, makarasana, matsyasana, vajrasana, ardha padmasana, shavasana, pavana-muktasana, and simple pranayama like anuloma-viloma and abdominal breathing are advantageous. Water treatments for hypertension include hot foot or leg bath for ten minutes, hot compress over the heart replacing it as bath cools down. Persons suffering from hypertension must ensure at least eight hours of soothing sleep, because proper rest is an important part of the treatment. Most important of all, the patient must avoid over-straining, worries, tension, anger and haste. He must try to be jolly and develop a contented mind. The natural treatment may take sometime but it is the safest and best way to get rid of this disease.

Chapter 11

Insomnia

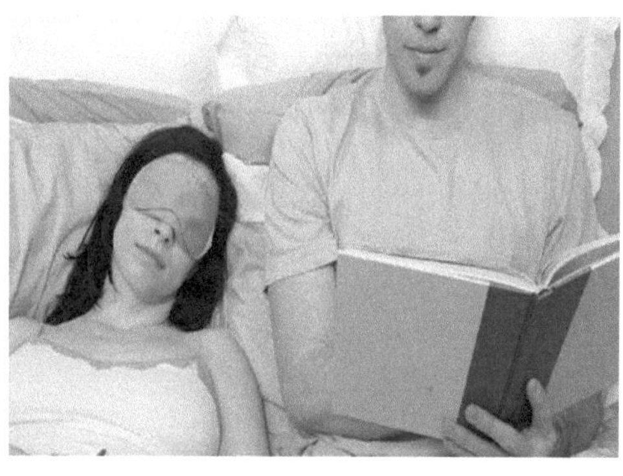

In the natural cure of insomnia, early to bed and early to rise is a good rule. Two hours of sleep before midnight are more beneficial than four after. Research has shown that people with chronic insomnia almost invariably marked deficiencies of such key nutrients as B-complex vitamins, and vitamin C and D as also calcium, magnesium, manganese, potassium and zinc. The sleep mechanism is unable to function efficiently unless each of these nutrients is present in adequate amounts in the diet. A balanced diet with simple modifications in the eating pattern will go a long way in the treatment and cure of insomnia. Such a diet should exclude white flour products, sugar and its products, tea, coffee, chocolate, cola drinks, alcohol, foods containing additives that are chemicals for preserving, colouring and flavouring, too much use of salt and strong condiments.

In the modified eating pattern, breakfast should consist of fresh and dried fruits, whole cereals, seeds and yogurt. Of the two main meals, one should comprise a large mixed salad and the other should be protein-based. A cup of milk sweetened with honey at bedtime is helpful as the amino-acid tryptophan contained in milk induces sleep. Any attempt to force sleep only drives it further away. It is better to redirect the mind with soft music or light reading. While going to bed, the patient should visualise a blank black wall occupying the entire field of vision. During the night, the position of the arms and legs should be changed regularly and a healthy sleeper usually shifts from one side to the other a number of times in the course of the night.

Controlled breathing is also a great help in inducing sleep. The method is to lie on one's side in bed, and then take three deep breaths expanding the abdomen entirely. Then breath should be held as long as possible. While holding breath, carbon dioxide accumulates in the body and induces natural sleep. Regular, active exercising during the day and mild exercise at bedtime enhances the quantity and the quality of sleep. Exercise stimulates the elimination of lactic acid from the body which correlates with stress and muscular tension. Regular exercise also produces hormonal changes which are advantageous to the body and to the sleep pattern. Walking, jogging, skipping, swimming are all ideal exercises. Vigorous exercise should, however, be avoided at night as this can be over-stimulating.

Yoga asanas helps a majority of cases of insomnia in two ways. Firstly, yoga treatment helps tone up the glandular, respiratory and nervous system. Secondly, yoga also gives physical and mental relaxation as a safety value for one's disturbing problems. The traditional yoga asanas which are effective for insomnia patients are shirsana, sarvangasana, paschimottanasana, uttanasan, viparita karani and shavasana. Hydrotherapy is also effective in treatment of insomnia. Along with the various measures for the treatment of insomnia, all efforts should be made to eliminate as many stress factors as possible. The steps in this direction should include regular practice of any relaxation method or meditation technique, cultivating the art of doing things slowly (particularly activities like eating, walking and talking), cultivating a creative hobby and spending some time daily on this, avoiding working against unrealistic targets and completing one task before starting another.

Chapter 12

Leucoderma

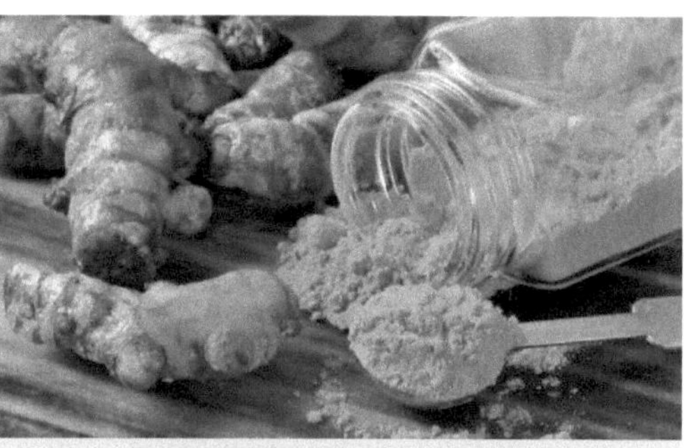
Turmeric For Leucoderma

In naturopathy, the natural treatment of leucoderma involves in flushing out the toxins from the system. This measure enables the healing power within the body to assert itself, and produce normalcy. To begin with, the patient should take on a fast on juices for about a week. In this regimen, he or she should take fruit or vegetable juices, diluted with water every two or three hours from 8.00 a.m. to 8.00 p.m. The bowels should be cleansed on a daily basis with warm water during this period. After the juice fast, the patient may adopt a restricted diet consisting of fresh fruits, raw or steamed vegetables and whole meal bread or chappatis. Curd and milk may be added to this diet after a few days.

The patient may from then on gradually embark upon a well-balanced diet of seeds, nuts and grains, vegetables and fruits. The large proportion of the diet should consist of raw foods. Seeds and beans such as alfalfa, and soyabeans can be sprouted. This diet may be supplemented with cold-pressed vegetable oils, honey and yeast. Juice fasting may be repeated at intervals of two months. The patient should avoid tea, coffee, alcoholic beverages and all condiments and highly flavoured dishes. He or she should also avoid sugar, white flour products, denatured cereals like polished rice and pearled barley and tinned or bottled foods.

Few home remedies have been found useful in the treatment of leucoderma. The best known of such remedies is the use of seeds of psoralea, known as babchi in Hindi. Seeds should be steeped in the juice of ginger or cow's urine for three days. The seeds should then be rubbed with hands to remove their husks, dried in the shade and powdered. One gram of this powder should be taken every day with fresh milk for forty days continuously. The ground seeds should also be applied to the white spots. Babchi seeds, combined with tamarind seeds, are also of use. Equal quantity of both the seeds should be steeped in water for three to four days. They should then be shelled and dried in the shade. They should be ground into paste and applied to the white patches for a week. If the application of this paste causes itching or the white spots become red and a fluid being to ooze out, it should be discontinued.

Another functional remedy for leucoderma is red clay found by the river side or on hill slopes. The clay should be mixed in ginger juice and applied over the white spots once a day. The copper contained in the clay seems to bring back skin pigmentation and ginger juice serves as a milk stimulant, facilitating increased blood flow to the spots. Drinking water kept overnight in a copper vessel also helps. A paste made from the seeds of the radish is helpful in treating Leucoderma. About thirty five grams of these seeds should be powdered in vinegar and applied on the white patches. For better results, seeds should be delicately pounded, mixed with a little white arsenic and soaked in vinegar at night. After two hours, when leaves appear, it should be rubbed on the Leucoderma patches.

The use of turmeric and mustard oil is also considered valuable in the treatment of leucoderma. About five hundred grams of turmeric should be pounded and soaked in eight kilograms of water at night. It should be heated in the morning till only one kg of water is left. It should then be strained and mixed with five hundred grams of mustard oil. This mixture should be heated till only the oil is left. It should be applied on white patches every morning and evening for a few months.

Chapter 13

Nepthritis

In naturopathy, the natural remedy of nephritis is fasting. The patient should resort to juice fasting for seven to ten days till the acute symptoms subside. Mostly vegetable juices such as carrot, celery and cucumber should be used during this period. A warm water enema should be taken each day while fasting, to cleanse the bowels of the toxic matter being thrown off by the self-cleansing process resulting from the fast. After the juice fast, the patient may adopt an all-fruit diet for four to five days. Juicy fruits such as apples, grapes, oranges, pears, peaches and pineapples should be taken during this period at five-hourly intervals. After the all-fruit diet, the patient may adopt fruits and milk diet. In this regimen, milk, preferably raw goat's milk may be added to the fruit diet for further seven days.

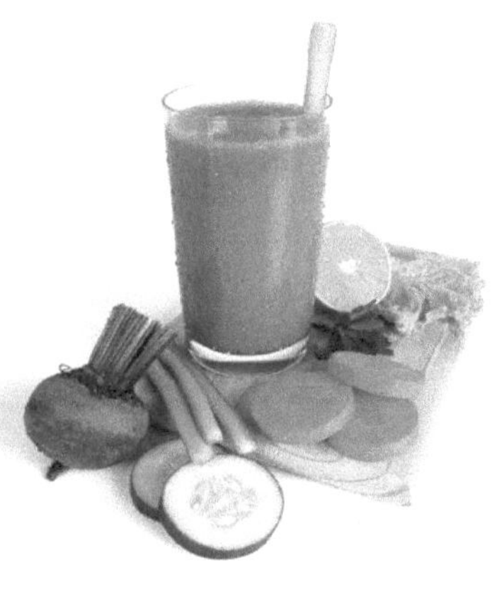

Thereafter the patient may slowly embark upon a well- balanced low protein vegetarian diet, with emphasis on fresh fruits and raw and cooked vegetables. In case of chronic Nepthritis a short juice fast for three days may be undertaken. Subsequently, a week or ten days may be spent on a controlled diet. In this regimen, oranges or orange juice may be taken for breakfast. Lunch may consist of a salad of raw vegetables which are in season, and dinner may comprise one or two vegetables, steamed in their own juices and a few nuts. The patient should avoid vegetables containing large quantities of oxalic acid such as spinach and rhubarb. Chocolate and cocoa also contain oxalic acid and must not be used. Garlic, asparagus, parsley, watercress, cucumber and celery are excellent vegetables. The best fruits are papaya and bananas. Both have a healing effect on kidneys. A small amount of soured milk and home- made cottage cheese can be included in the diet.

All salt should be eliminated from the diet. Five or six small meals should be taken in preference to a few large ones. A glassful of carrot juice mixed with tablespoonful of honey and a teaspoonful of fresh lime juice is a very successful home remedy for Nepthritis. It should be taken every day early in the morning before breakfast. Bananas are also valuable in Nepthritis because of their low protein and salt content and high carbohydrates content. In this condition, a diet of bananas only should be taken for three or four days, consuming eight to nine bananas a day. Smoking and drinking, where habitual, must be totally given up. Studies have shown that smoking impairs kidney function. The patient should avoid white bread, sugar, cakes, pastries, puddings, and refined cereals, greasy, heavy or fried foods. He should also avoid tea, coffee, all flesh foods, condiments, pickles, and sauces.

All measures should be adopted to relieve the kidneys of work by escalating elimination through other channels. Hot Epsom salt bath should be taken every alternate day to encourage elimination through the skin as much as possible. Fresh air and outdoor exercises will be of great advantage in all cases of nepthritis and where possible, the patient should have a walk for at least three kilometers once or twice on a daily basis. The sufferer from chronic nNepthritis should never exert himself when doing anything. He should avoid all hurry and excitement.

Chapter 14

Piles

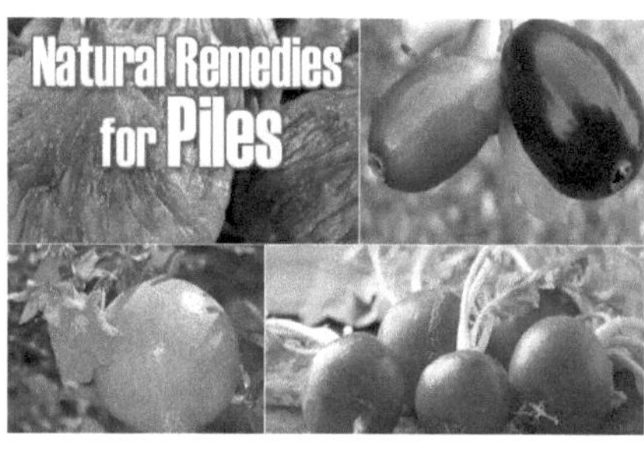

In the natural remedy for piles, the patient should adopt an all-fruit diet for at least seven days. After the all-fruit diet, the patient may adopt a diet of natural foods aimed at securing soft stools. The most vital food remedy for piles is dry figs. Three or four figs should be soaked overnight in water after cleansing them methodically in hot water. They should be taken the first thing in the morning along with water in which they were soaked. They should also be taken in the evening in a similar manner. This therapy should be continued for three or four weeks. The tiny seeds of the fruit possess an exceptional quality of stimulating peristalic movements of intestines. This facilitates easy evacuation of faeces and keeps the alimentary canal clean.

Mango seeds are regarded as an efficient medication for bleeding piles. The seeds should be collected during the mango season, dried in the shade and powdered and kept stored for use as medicine. It should be given in doses of about one and a half gram to two grams with or without honey. The jambul fruit is another effective food remedy for bleeding piles. The fruit should be taken with salt every morning for two or three months in its season. White radish is considered extremely valuable in the treatment of piles. White radish well ground into a paste in milk can also be beneficial applied over inflamed pile masses to ease pain and swelling. The patient should drink at least six to eight glasses of water a day. He should avoid straining to pass a stool. Cold water treatment helps the veins to shrink and tones up their walls. Other water treatments advantageous in curing piles include cold perennial douche and cold compress applied to the rectal area for an hour before bed time. A patient with piles must make an all out effort to tone up the entire system.

Exercise plays an important remedial role in this condition. Movements which exercise the abdominal muscles will improve circulation in the rectal region and relieve congestion. Outdoor exercises such as walking and swimming are excellent methods of building up general health. Yogic kriyas like jalneti and vamandhouti and asanas such as sarvangasana, viparit karani, halasana, gomukhasana are also useful.

Chapter 15

Rheumatism

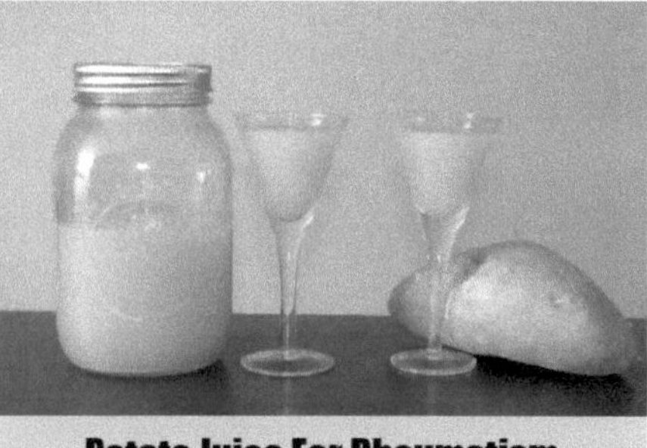
Potato Juice For Rheumatism

In the natural cure of Rheumatism, the patient should be put on a short fast of orange juice and water for three or four days. While fasting, the bowels should be cleansed in the course of warm water enema. After the juice fast, the patient should be placed on a restricted diet for fourteen days. In this regimen, orange or grapefruit may be taken for breakfast; lunch may consist of a raw salad of any vegetables in season, with raisins, prunes, figs or dates; and for dinner, one or two steamed vegetables such as spinach, cabbage, carrots, turnips, cauliflower, etc., and a few nuts or some sweet fruit may be taken. Thereafter, the patient may steadily commence a well balanced diet of three basic food groups, namely (i) seeds, nuts and grains (ii) vegetables and (iii) fruits.

In case of chronic rheumatism, the patient may be placed on an all-fruit diet for four or five days. In this course of therapy, he should have three meals a day of fresh, juicy fruits such as apples, grapes, peaches, pears, oranges, pineapples and grapefruit. He may subsequently adopt a well balanced diet. The patient should take ripe fruits and fresh vegetables in abundance. The foods which should be avoided are meat, fish, white bread, sugar, refined cereals, rich, indigestible and highly seasoned foods tea, coffee, alcohol, sauces, pickles and condiments. Raw potato juice is regarded as an exceptional food medication for rheumatism. One or two teaspoonful of the juice pressed out of mashed raw potato should be taken before meals. This will help eliminate an acid condition and relieve rheumatism.

Celery is another useful food remedy for rheumatism. A fluid extract of the seeds is more powerful than the raw vegetable. This also has a tonic action on the stomach and kidneys. Five to ten drops of this fluid should be taken in hot water before meals. Powdered seeds can be used as a condiment. Lemons are also valuable and the juice of two or three lemons may be taken each day. Other helpful methods in the treatment of rheumatism are application of radiant heat and hot packs to the affected parts, a hot tub bath, cabinet steam bath, dry friction and a sponge bath. Hot Epsom salt baths are also beneficial and should be taken twice a week for three months in case of chronic rheumatism and once weekly thereafter. Fresh air, deep breathing and light outdoor exercises are also advantageous. Dampness and cold should be avoided.

Chapter 16

Impotence

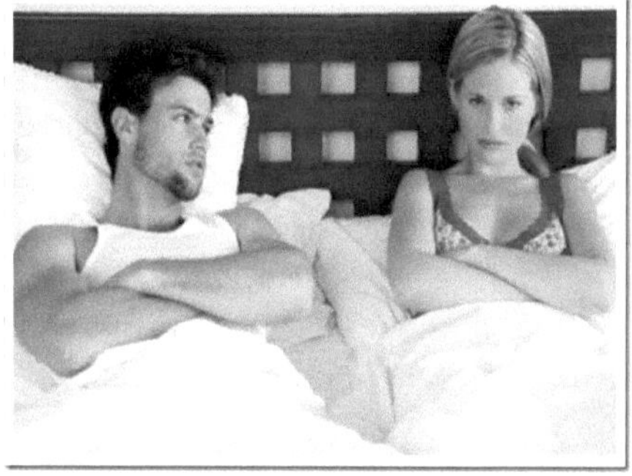

In the natural cure of impotence, diet is of supreme significance. To begin with, the patient should adopt an exclusive fresh fruit diet from five to seven days. In this regimen, he can have three meals a day, at five hourly intervals, of fresh juicy fruits such as grapes, oranges, apples, pears, peaches, pineapple and melon. The bowels should be cleansed on a daily basis during this period with a warm-water enema. After the all-fruit diet, the patient may steadily embark upon a balanced diet of seeds, nuts and grains, vegetables and fruits, with generous use of rejuvenating foods such as whey, soured milks, particularly made from goat's milk, millet, garlic, honey, cold-pressed vegetable oils and brewer's yeast. The patient should avoid smoking, alcohol, tea, coffee and all processed, canned, refined and denatured foods, especially white sugar and white flour and products made from them.

Certain foods are considered highly advantageous in the treatment of impotence. The most important of these is garlic. It is a natural and harmless aphrodisiac. Onion is another important aphrodisiac food. It stands second only to garlic. It increases libido and strengthens the reproductory organs. The white variety of onion, is however, more useful for this purpose. Carrot is also considered useful in impotence. For better results, carrot should be taken with a half-boiled egg dipped in a tablespoonful of honey once daily for a month or two. This recipe increases sex stamina by releasing sex hormones and strengthens the sexual plexus. It is for this reason that carrot halwa, prepared according to Unani specifications is considered a very effectual tonic to improve sexual strength.

The lady's finger is another great tonic for improving sexual vigour. It has been mentioned in ancient Indian literature that the persons who take five to ten grams of root powder of this vegetable with milk and `misri` on a daily basis will never lose sexual vigour. Black raisins are also useful for restoration of sexual dynamism. They should be boiled with milk after washing them thoroughly in lukewarm water. This will make them swollen and sweet. Eating of such raisins should be followed by the use of milk. Starting with thirty grams of raising with 200 ml. of milk, three times daily, the quantity of raisin should be slowly increased to 50 grams each time. A vigorous massage all over the body is highly favourable in the healing of impotence as it will restore the muscular vigour which is vital for nervous energy. Every attempt should be made to build up the general health level to the highest degree and fresh air and outdoor exercise are indispensable to the success of the treatment. Yoga asanas such as dhanurasana, sarvangasana and halasana are also extremely beneficial.

Chapter 17

Tonsillitis

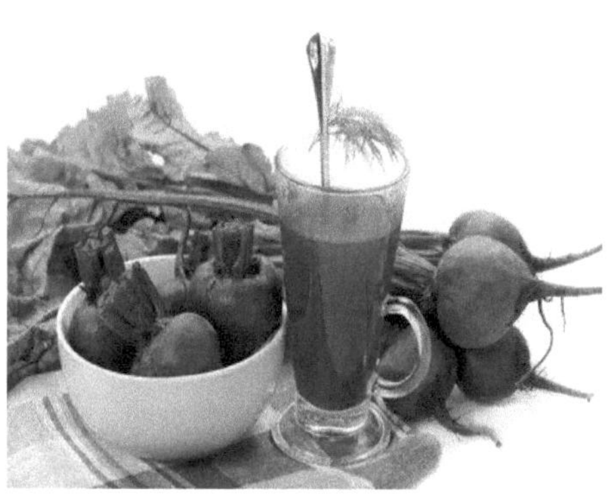

Natural cure of tonsillitis prescribes an appropriate diet where the patient should begin with fast for three to five days by which time the severe symptoms would settle. Nothing but water and orange juice should be taken for this period of time. The bowels should be cleansed on a daily basis with a lukewarm water enema during the period of fasting. A cold pack should be applied to the throat at two hourly intervals at the time of the day. The procedure is to wring out some linen material in cold water, wrap it two or three times around the throat and envelop it with some flannelling. The throat may be gargled a number of times daily with neat lemon juice. Gargle made from the fenugreek seeds is very helpful in severe cases.

A hot Epsom salt bath taken every day or every other day will also be advantageous. After the acute symptoms of tonsillitis are over, the patient should take up an all fruit diet for further three or four days. In this course of therapy, three meals of fresh, juicy fruits such as apples, pineapple, peaches, grapes, grapefruit, oranges, pears and melon may be taken. The juice of fresh pineapple is most valuable in all throat afflictions of this kind.

After the all-fruit diet the patient may gradually embark upon a well balanced diet on the following lines:

- **Breakfast:** Fresh fruits, or grated raw carrot or any other raw salad, and milk. Prunes or other dried fruits may be added, if desired.

- **Lunch:** Steamed vegetables, as obtainable and whole wheat chappatis. Vegetables likes bitter gourd and fenugreek are in particular advantageous.
- **Dinner:** A good sized raw salad of vegetables as available sprouts seeds as alfalfa seeds, whole meal bread and butter or cottage cheese.

Raw vegetable juices are also very functional in the cure of tonsillitis. Juices of carrot, beet and cucumber taken individually or in combination are in particular of assistance. The daily dry friction and hip bath as well as breathing and other exercises should all form part of the daily health regime. A hot Epsom salts bath once or twice a week can also be taken on a regular basis with beneficial results. Tonsillitis can be successfully treated by the natural methods outlined above. Surgery for the removal of the tonsils is required only in very rare cases, when tonsils are critically diseased.

Chapter 18

Varicose Veins

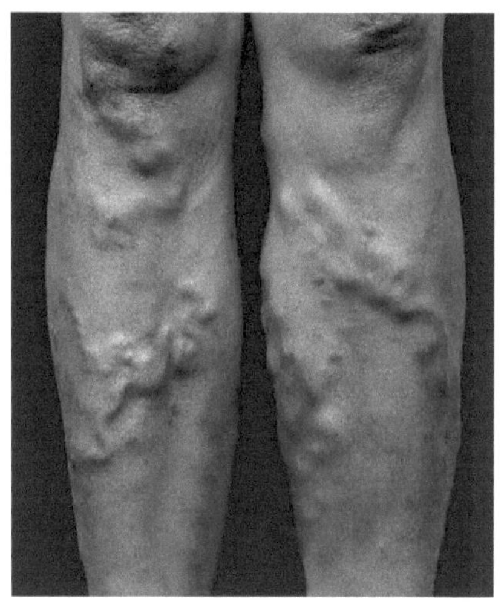

In the natural remedy for varicose veins, the patients should, in the commencement of the treatment, be put on a juice fast for four or five days or on all-fruit diet for seven to ten days. A lukewarm water enema should be administered on a daily basis during this phase to cleanse the bowels and measures should be taken to keep away from constipation. After the juice fast or all the fruit diet, the patient should take on a restricted diet plan. In this course of therapy, oranges or orange and lemon juice may be taken for breakfast. The midday meal may consist of a raw salad or any of the vegetables in the season with olive oil and lemon juice dressing. Steamed vegetables such as spinach, cabbage, turnips, cauliflower, carrots, and raisins, figs or dates may be taken in the evening. No bread or potatoes or other starchy food should be included in this diet, or otherwise the whole effect of the diet will be lost.

Subsequent to the restricted diet, the patient may little by little embark upon a well balanced diet with emphasis on grains, seeds, nuts, vegetables and fruits. All condiments, alcoholic drinks, coffee, strong tea, white flour products, white sugar, and white sugar products should be firmly avoided. A short fast or the all fruit diet for two or three days may be undertaken every month, depending on the improvement. Raw vegetables juices, chiefly carrot juice in combination with spinach juice, have proved extremely advantageous in the treatment of varicose veins. Certain nutrients, in particular vitamin E and C have also been found effective in the treatment of this disease. The alternate hot and cold hip bath is very valuable and should be taken on a daily basis. The affected parts should be sprayed with cold water or cold packs should be applied to them. A mud pack may be applied at night and allowed to remain until morning. A hot Epsom salt bath is also very valuable and should be taken twice a week.

Certain inverted yoga postures such as viparita karani, sarvagasana, and shirshashana are beneficial in the treatment of varicose veins as they drain the blood from the legs and lessen pressure on the veins. They help to relax the muscles and allow the blood freely in and out of the lower extremities. Padmasana, vajrasana, gomukhasana and salabhasana are also advantageous for the cure.

Chapter 19

Menopausal Problems

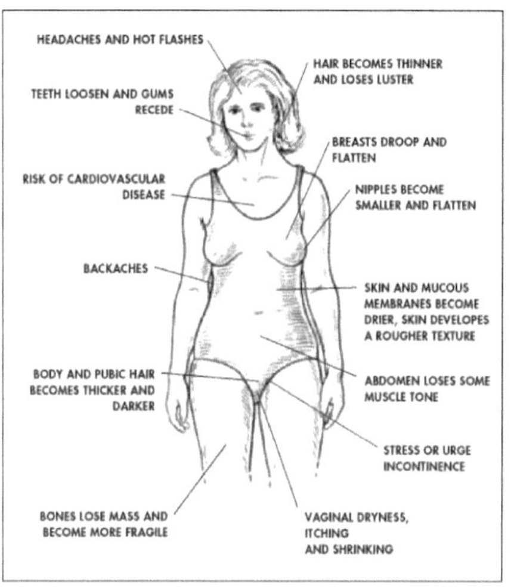

In naturopathy the natural cure for menopausal problems can be dealt with a proper diet and a right mental attitude. Although menopause cannot be avoided, it can be postponed for as long as ten to fifteen years. The body of a woman needs a meticulous cleansing and for this reason, she should undertake a course of natural health building treatment. Diet is of supreme importance in such a scheme of treatment. In fact the problems at menopause are often much more stern than that at puberty largely because the diet has been scarce for many years prior to its onset, in many nutrients such as protein, calcium, magnesium, vitamins D, E and pantothenic acid.

The diet of the patient should be made up from three basic food groups, namely (i) seeds, nuts and grains (ii) vegetables and (iii) fruits. The importance should be on vitamin E-rich raw and sprouted seeds, unpasteurised high quality milk and home-made cottage cheese and an abundance of raw, organically grown fruits and vegetables. Ample of freshly made juices of fruits and vegetables in season should also be included in this diet. All processed and denatured foods, such as white sugar, white flour and all articles made with them, should be entirely eliminated. During menopause, the lack of ovarian hormones can result in a severe calcium deficiency. Vitamins D and F are also essential for assimilation of calcium.

During the menopause, the need for vitamin E soars ten to fifty times over that formerly required. Hot flashes, night sweats and other symptoms of menopause often fade away when 50 to 100 units of vitamin E are taken on a daily basis. The symptoms reappear rapidly if the vitamin is discontinued. Of late, it has become popular to take estrogen to prevent or postpone menopausal symptoms. Beet juice has been found very functional in menopausal disorders. It should be taken in small quantities of 60 to 90 ml at a time thrice a day. It has proved much more enduringly helpful than the degenerative effects of drugs or synthetic hormones. Carrot seeds have also been found valuable in menopausal tension. A teaspoonful of the seeds should be boiled in a glassful of cow's milk for about ten minutes and taken on a daily basis as a medicine.

Outdoor exercise, such as walking, swimming, jogging, horse-riding or cycling, is very important to postpone menopause. Other helpful measures in this direction are avoiding mental and emotional anxiety and worries especially worry about growing old, adequate sleep and relaxation and following all general rules of maintaining a high level of health. The healthier a woman is, the fewer menopausal symptoms she will experience. The menopause can be made a pleasurable affair by building bodily health and a rational mental attitude.

Chapter 20

Vaginitis

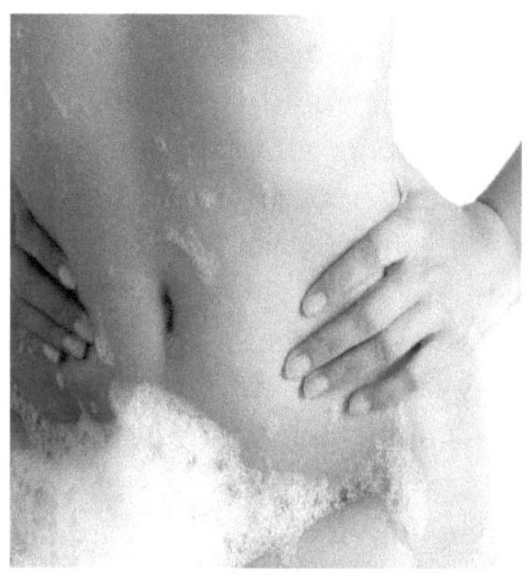

Natural remedy for vaginitis involves the maintenance of a hygienic condition which is considered as the most important factor in the treatment. Another significant factor is the diet. The patient should be made to fast for three or five days. The fasting period may be extended depending on the condition. During this period, the patient may take juices of lemon and other sub acidic fruits. This will give the system a chance to redirect its vital energies to check inflammation and infection. After the juice fasting, the patient may take on restricted diet, consisting of raw vegetable salads, fruits and sprouts. This will ensure minimal mucous secretions. This restricted diet should be sustained for ten to fifteen days. It will help lessen inflammatory conditions. Boiled vegetables which are effortlessly digestible and wheat chappatis may be added slowly to this diet. Later, rice, vegetable soup or butter milk may be taken for lunch and an uncooked diet for dinner.

The patient should keep away from coffee, tea and other stimulants as well as sugar, fried and refined foods.

Water therapy plays a significant role in the cure of Vaginitis. The patient should be given an enema with lukewarm neem water to cleanse the bowels and avoid the constipation which increases the toxemic condition, inflammation and infection in the genital organs. For general cleansing and elimination of purulent vaginal discharge, neem water vaginal douche at 35 o C - 40 o C followed by cold douche will be extremely helpful. In constant cases, cold vaginal irritation provides respite. This treatment is best administered with a fountain syringe, containing water. The syringe should be placed two or three feet above the patient and water injected into the vagina. The patient should lie upon her back, with hips elevated and water should flow out of the vaginal canal. A decoction of the herb chebulic myrobalan has proved very functional for vaginal irritation and inflammation. It should be used as an external douche to wash the vulvar parts. When there is a thick white discharge, washing the part with decoction made with neem leaves and chebulic myrobalan fruits will be of great help.

A reasonably prolonged cold hip bath accompanied with a hot foot bath is also helpful. The level of cold water must be thirty four inches in height. The patient should sit in the tub in such a manner that legs remain out of the tub. This bath can be given for twenty to thirty minutes. Another method of treatment considered valuable is the wet girdle pack for about an hour. For this treatment, thin cotton underwear and thick or woolen underwear are required. The thin underwear should be wrung in cold water and worn by the patient. The thick dry underwear should be worn above the wet underwear. If the patient feels chill, she should be covered with a blanket. This treatment helps lessen inflammation. A cold douche on the perennial region for ten to fifteen minutes twice a day helps reduce Vaginitis. A mud pack on the abdomen for ten minutes twice on a daily basis also helps diminish inflammation.

Chromotherapy or colour therapy can also be used in the treatment of this disease. Blue light treatment given to the afflicted region for an hour accompanied with vaginal irrigation using green coloured charged water helps reduce the infection. After recovery, it is necessary to adopt proper eating habits and hygienic living conditions. Appropriate rest and exercise are also significant.

Chapter 21

Hysteria

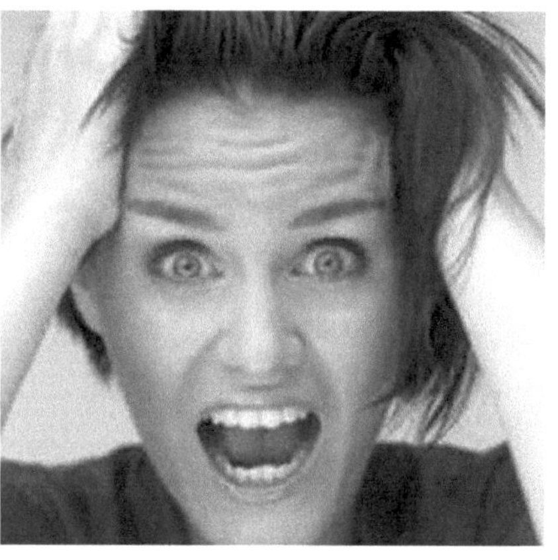

In the Natural Remedy for Hysteria, the treatment is directed toward both the body and the mind since the causes of hysteria are both physical and mental. The measures on the physical side should include a well ordered hygienic style of living, a nourishing and balanced diet, sufficient mental and physical rest, daily exercise , agreeable, occupation, fresh air, normal hours of eating and sleeping, regulation of the bowels and wholesome companionship with others. On the mental plane, the patient should be taught self-control and educated in optimistic thinking.

In the majority cases of hysteria, it is desirable for the patient to start treatment by adopting an all fruit diet for a number of days. She should have fresh juicy fruits such as orange, grapefruit, apple, grapes, papaya and pineapple during this period. The all-fruit diet should be followed by an exclusive milk diet for about a month. Most hysteria patients are significantly run down and the milk diet will help build better blood and nourish the nerves. If the full milk diet is not suitable, a diet of milk and fruits may be adopted. The patient, may, therefore, steadily embark upon a well balanced diet of seeds, nuts and grains. The patient should avoid alcohol, tobacco, tea, coffee, white sugar and white flour and products made from them.

Jambul fruit, known as jamun in the vernacular, is considered a useful home medication for hysteria. Women suffering from hysteria should take three hundred grams of this fruit on an empty stomach. This treatment should be continued for two weeks. Honey is regarded as another effective remedy for hysteria. Two of the main causes of hysteria are irregularity of the menstrual cycle and insanity. Honey is very useful for both these conditions. It causes good bleeding during the cycle, cleans the uterus, tones up the brain and the uterine musculature and keeps the body temperature at a normal level. It is prudent to use honey on a regular basis and increase the quantity after the first start. It will bring down body temperature thus preventing further fits.

Exercise and outdoor games are essential in the prevention and cure of hysteria. They take the mind away from one`s self and stimulate cheerfulness. Yoga asanas which are useful in hysteria are matsyasana, sarvangasana, dhanurasana, halasana, bhujangasana, salabhasana, paschimotanasana, yogamudra and shavasana. Weak patients, who are not able to take much active exercise, may be given massage three or four times a week. Other measures functional in the treatment of hysteria are air and sun baths. They are calming and at the same time invigorating to the nerves. Daily cool baths are also an outstanding tonic. Suitable physical activity must be balanced with sufficient rest and sleep.

In a genuine hysterical attack, the most successful means of interrupting the paroxysm is the application of cold water in some form to the head and spine. Either the cold water may be poured or cold pack or ice pack may be applied to the hand and back of the neck. If this cannot be done, cold water may be splashed on the face. The patient should be provided with abundance of fresh air and some of her clothing should be removed to assist easy breathing and to expose the skin to fresh air. In a violent seizure of hysteria, pressure on the ovaries often checks the attack. Following an attack the patient should have rest, tranquility, darkness and if possible, sleep until the lost energy has been progressively recovered.

Chapter 22

Dermatitis

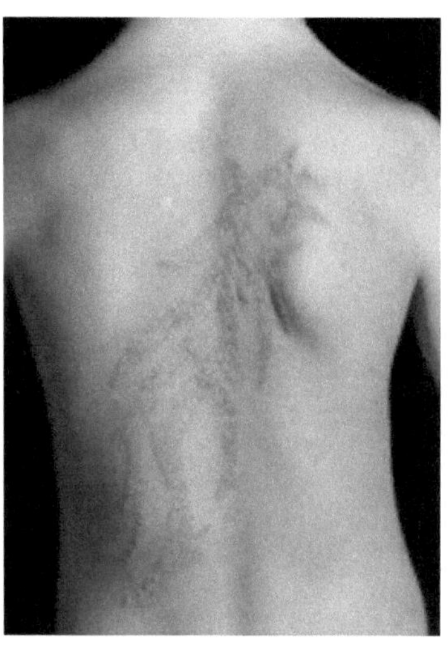

Natural Remedy for Dermatitis prescribes the patient to commence the treatment by adopting an all-fruit diet for at least a week. In this course of therapy, he should take three meals a day of juicy fruits such as orange, pineapple, grapes, apple and papaya at five hourly intervals. Subsequent to an exclusive fruit diet, patient may adopt a restricted diet for ten days. In this course of therapy, breakfast may comprise orange juice or grapefruit. Raw salad, consisting of vegetables available in season, with raisins, figs or dates may be taken for lunch and dinner may consist of steamed vegetables such as carrots, turnips, spinach, and cabbage, cauliflower, along with a few nuts or fresh fruit. Mild puddings and desserts such as jellies, jams and pastries, all condiments, white sugar, and white flour and products made from them, tea, coffee and other stimulating drinks should all be avoided.

Following the restricted diet, the patient should steadily embark upon a well balanced diet, which consists of seeds, nuts and grains, vegetables and fruits. The emphasis should be on fresh fruits and raw vegetables. In case of a severe situation, the patient should embark on a fast on fruit or vegetable juices for three to five days. This may be followed by a restricted diet for ten to fifteen days. Further fasts and a period on restricted diet at intervals may be adopted after the recommencement of a normal diet. The lukewarm water enema should be used on a daily basis to cleanse the bowels during the first week of treatment and subsequently as necessary. Epsom salts baths may be taken two or three times a week. The affected areas may also be bathed twice on a daily basis in hot water with Epsom salts. The patient should keep away from white sugar, refined carbohydrates, tea, coffee, and other denatured foods. He should make liberal use of fruits and vegetable juices. No medicines of any kind should be used. In case of trouble due to external causes, the most helpful treatment consists of applying a mixture of baking soda (bicarbonate of soda) and olive oil.

The patient should take on moderate physical exercise, preferably simple yoga asanas after the fast is completed and the start of the restricted diet. Exercise is one of the most valuable means for purifying the blood and for preventing toxaemia. The patient should also have sufficient physical and mental rest and fresh air. He should stay away from exposure to cold, and adopt regular hours of eating sleeping.

Chapter 23

Malaria

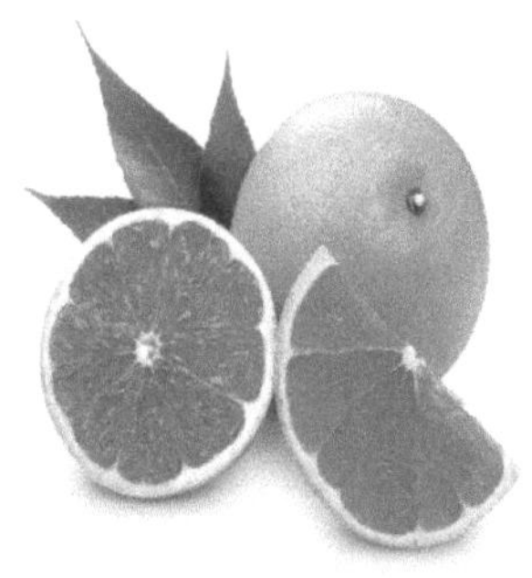

In the natural remedy for malaria, diet is of supreme importance. In the beginning of the treatment the patient should keep a fast on orange juice and water for seven to fifteen days depending on the severity of the fever. The tepid water enema should be administered on a daily basis during this period to cleanse the bowels. After the fever has subsided, the patient should be placed on an exclusive fresh fruit diet for more three days. In this course of therapy, he should take three meals a day, at five hourly intervals, of fresh, juicy fruits, like grapefruit, apple, pineapple, oranges, grapes, mango and papaya. Milk may be added to the fruit diet after this period and this diet may be continued for a further few days.

Subsequently, the patient may embark upon a well balanced diet of natural foods consisting of seeds, nuts and grains. The patient should stay away from strong tea, coffee, refined and processed foods, fried foods, condiments, sauces, pickles, white sugar, white flour, and all products made from them. He should also avoid all meats, alcoholic drinks and smoking. The best way to lessen temperature naturally, during the course of fever, is by means of the cold pack, which can be applied to the whole body. This pack is made by wringing out a sheet or other large square piece of linen material in cold water, wrapping it right round the body and legs of the patient (twice round would be best) and then covering from top to bottom with a small blanket or similar warm material. This pack should be applied every three hours during the day while temperature is high and kept on for an hour or so. Hot water bottles may be applied to the feet and also against the sides of the body.

Certain home remedies have been found advantageous in the cure of malaria. One such remedy is the use of grapefruit. This substance can be extracted from the fruits by boiling a quarter of the grapefruit and straining its pulp. Lime and lemon are beneficial in the treatment of quarter type of malaria fever. About three grams of lime should be dissolved in about 60 ml. of water and juice of one lemon added to it. This water should be taken before the onset of the fever. Cinnamon is regarded as a successful cure for all types of colds, as well as malaria. It should be crudely powdered and boiled in a glass of water with a pinch of pepper powder and honey. This can be used constructively as a medication in malaria. Alum (phitkari) is also useful in malaria. It should be roasted over a hot plate and powdered. It should be taken about four hours before the expected attack and every two hours after it. This will give great respite to the patient.

The preventive facet in malaria is as important as the curative one. The best way to defend against malaria is to take on all measures required for preventing mosquito bites. For this purpose, it is very important to maintain cleanliness of surroundings, environmental sanitation and to eradicate stretches of stagnant water. As the mosquito generally perches itself on the walls of the house, after biting a person, it would be advisable to spray the walls with insecticides. The leaves of the holy basil (tulsi) are considered valuable in the prevention of malaria. An infusion of some leaves can be taken on a daily basis for this purpose. The juice of about eleven grams of tulsi leaves mixed with three grams of black pepper, powder, can be taken beneficially in the cold stage of the malarial fever. This will check the severity of the disease.

Chapter 24

Measles

Natural remedy for measles requires that the patient should be given juices of fresh fruits like orange and lemon on a regular basis. This is adequate as the patient suffers from lack of appetite during this period. He should be kept in a well ventilated room. As light has a damaging effect upon the eyes during measles, because of the weakened condition of the external eye tissues, the patient should have his eyes shaded or the room should have subdued light. The cure should aim at bringing down the temperature and eliminating the toxins from the system. This can be achieved by administration of warm water enema every morning, application of mud packs on the abdomen twice a day in the morning and evening and repeated application of chest packs.

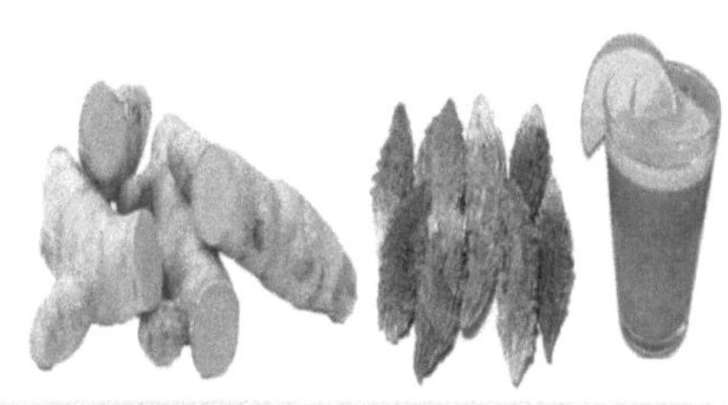

Turmeric And Bitter Gourd Juice For Measles

Tepid water baths can be given every day to ease itching. Addition of extracts of neem leaves to this water will prove advantageous. As the condition improves, the patient can be placed on an all fruit diet for a further few days. Subsequently he may be allowed to gradually embark upon a well balanced diet. Certain home remedies have been found beneficial in the treatment of measles. The most helpful amongst these is the use of orange. When the digestive power of the body is critically hampered, the patient suffers from intense toxaemia and the lack of saliva coats his tongue and often destroys his thirst for water as well as his desire for food. The agreeable flavour of orange juice helps to a great extent in overcoming these drawbacks. Orange juice is the most ideal liquid food in this disease.

The juice of lemon is another medication. It also makes an efficient thirst-quenching drink in measles. Turmeric (haldi) is beneficial in the treatment of measles. Raw roots of turmeric should be dried in the sun and ground to a fine powder. This powder, mixed with a few drops of honey and the juice of a few bitter gourd leaves, should be given to the patient afflicted from measles. Powdered liquorice (mulethi) has been found valuable in relieving the cough, typical of measles. The use of barley (Jau) water has proved useful in case of troublesome cough in measles. This water should be taken regularly sweetened with the newly drawn oil of sweet almonds. Children having measles should not be allowed to mix with others. They should be given absolute rest. Hygienic condition along with the above mentioned treatment will lead to speedy recuperation. Medications should be strictly avoided.

Chapter 25

Throat

Natural remedy for sore throat requires that the patient should fast on orange juice and water for three to five days, depending on the severity of the condition. He should take orange juice diluted with tepid water every two or three hours from 8 a.m. to 8 p.m. during this period. The bowels should be cleansed on a daily basis with lukewarm water enema. This should be done twice daily in more serious cases. A wet pack should be applied to the throat at two hourly intervals during the day, and also one at night. The procedure is to wring out some linen material in cold water, wrap two or three times round the effected part, and cover with some flanner. The throat may be gargled more than a few times with warm water mixed with a little salt. A hot Epsom salt bath, taken on a daily basis during this period, will be extremely advantageous.

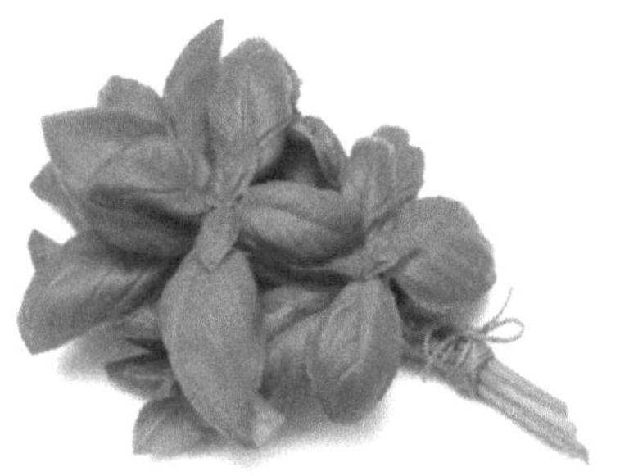

Basil For Sore Throat

When the more severe symptoms settle, the patient may take on an all fruit diet for three or four further days, taking three meals a day of juicy fruits such as orange, apple, pineapple and papaya at five hourly intervals. Subsequently he may slowly but surely adopt a well balanced diet, with emphasis on seeds, nuts and grains, raw vegetables and fresh fruits. The daily dry friction and deep breathing and other exercises should form part of the daily health schedule. Certain home remedies have been found to be valuable in the treatment of sore throat. One such remedy is use of mango (aam) bark which is very effective in sore throat and other throat disorders. Its fluid can be applied locally with beneficial results. It can also be used as a throat gargle. The herb belleric myrobian (bahera) is another valuable medication for sore throat. A mixture of the pulp of the fruit, salt, long pepper (pipli) and honey should be administered in the treatment of this condition. The fried fruit, roasted after covering it with wheat flour, is also a popular remedy for sore throat.

Betel leaves (pan - ka -patta) have proved helpful in the treatment of this disease. The leaves should be applied locally for obtaining relief. The fruit of the betel tree, mixed with honey, can also be taken beneficially to relieve irritating throat cough. The bishop`s weed (ajwain) is important in treating sore throat. An infusion of the seeds mixed with common salt can be used beneficially as a gargle in acute condition caused by colds. The spice cinnamon (dalchini) is also regarded as a successful tonic for sore throat, resulting from cold. Coarsely powdered and boiled in a glass of water with a pinch of pepper powder and honey, it can be taken as a medication in the treatment of this condition. The oil of cinnamon, mixed with honey, also gives huge relief. A gargle prepared from fenugreek (methi) seeds has been found very efficient remedy for treating sore throat.

The leaves of the holy basil or tulsi have also been found advantageous in the treatment of this condition. The water boiled with basil leaves should be taken as a drink and also used as a gargle in sore throat. The patient should keep away from rapid changes in temperature like hot sun-shine to air conditioned rooms. He should stay away from cold and sore foods which may irritate his throat. To prevent the disease, a person should avoid touching tissues, handkerchief, towels or utensils used by the patients suffering from sore throat.

Chapter 26

Hair Fall

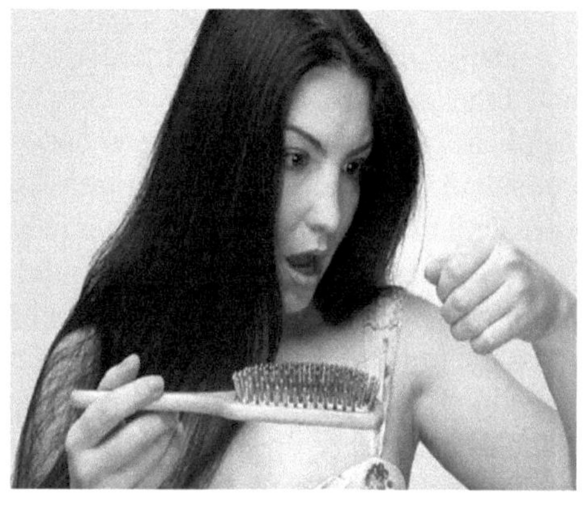

Natural remedy for hair fall depends largely on the intake of sufficient amount of vital nutrients in the daily diet. It is supplied by milk, buttermilk, eggs, cheese, yogurt, soyabean, meat and fish. A lack of vitamin A may cause the hair to be coarse and ugly. A shortage of some of the B vitamins, of iron, copper and iodine may cause hair disorders like falling of hair and untimely graying. Persons with a propensity to lose hair should thus take a well balanced and proper diet, made up of foods which in combination should supply all the necessary nutrients. It has been found that a diet which contains liberal quantities of (i) seeds, nuts and grains, (ii) vegetables and (iii) fruits would supply sufficient amounts of all the essential nutrients.

Each food group should more or less form the bulk of one of the three principal meals. These foods should, however, be supplemented with certain special foods such as milk, wheat germ, vegetable oils, honey, yeast and liver. A number of home remedies have been found functional in the prevention and treatment of the loss of the hair. The most successful among these remedies is a vigorous rubbing of the scalp with fingers after washing the hair with cold water. The scalp should be rubbed vigorously till it starts to tingle with the heat. It will make active the sebaceous glands and energise the circulation of blood in the affected area, making the hair grow healthy.

Amla oil, prepared by boiling dry pieces of amla in coconut oil, is considered an important hair tonic for enriching hair growth. A mixture of equal quantity of fresh amla juice and lime juice used as a shampoo stimulates hair growth and prevents hair loss. Lettuce (salad- ka- patta) is valuable in preventing hair loss through deficiencies. A concoction of lettuce and spinach juice is said to help the growth of hair if it is drunk to the extent of half a litre a day. The juice of alfalfa (lecerne) in combination with carrot and lettuce juice, taken on a daily basis also helps the growth of hair to a notable extent. The combination of these juices is rich in elements which are chiefly useful for the growth of hair. While preparing alfalfa juice, the leaves of the plant only may be used when it can be obtained fresh.

Daily application of refined coconut oil mixed with limewater and lime juice on the hair, prevents loss of hair and lengthens them. Application of the juice of green coriander leaves on the head is also considered advantageous. Amaranth, known as chaulai- ka- saag in the vernacular, is another valuable remedy. Application of its fresh leaf-juice helps the growth of the hair and keeps them soft. Mustard oil, boiled with henna leaves, is useful in healthy growth of hair. A regular massage of the head with this oil will produce abundant hair. One more valuable home medication for loss of hair is the application of coconut milk all over the scalp and massaging it into the hair loss. It will nourish the hair and encourage hair growth. The coconut milk is prepared by grinding the coconut shavings and squeezing it well.

Washing the hair with a paste of cooked black gram dal, (urad dal) and fenugreek (methi) lengthens the hair. A fine paste made from pigeon pea or red gram (arhar dal) can also be applied on a regular basis with beneficial results on bald patches. Regular use of castor oil as hair oil helps the abundant growth of the hair. Certain home remedies have also been found useful in case of patchy loss of hair. The seeds of lime and black pepper seeds, ground to get a fine paste, are one of the valuable remedies. This paste applied on the patches, has slightly irritant action. This increases blood circulation in the affected area and stimulates hair growth. The paste should be applied twice a day for a few weeks. Another practical remedy for patchy loss of hair is the paste of liquorice (mulethi) made by grinding the pieces in milk with a pinch of saffron. This paste should be applied over the bald patches in the night before going to bed.

Chapter 27

High Blood Cholesterol

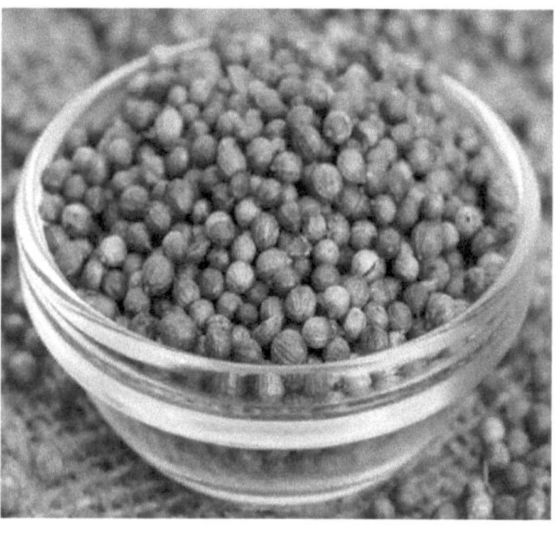

In naturopathy, the natural remedy for high blood cholesterol can be obtained by keeping away from foods rich in cholesterol and saturated fats. Diet is the most important factor in the cure. Cholesterol rich foods are bacon, beef, eggs, meats, cheese, butter, whole milk, virtually all foods of animal origin as well as two vegetable oils, namely coconut and palm, are high in saturated fats and these should be replaced by polyunsaturated fats such as corn, safflower, soyabeans and sesame oils which tend to lower the level of low density lipoproteins (LDL). There are mono saturated fats such as olive and peanut oils which have more or less neutral effect on the LDL level.

The quantity of fiber in the diet also influences the cholesterol levels and LDL cholesterol can be lowered by taking diets rich in fibers. The most important sources of dietary fiber are unprocessed wheat bran, whole cereals such as barley, wheat, rice, rye; legumes such as carrot, beet, potato, and turnips; fruits like mango and guava and green vegetables such as cabbage, lady's finger, lettuce and celery. Oat bran is in particular advantageous in lowering LDL cholesterol. Lecithin, also a fatty food substance and the most abundant of the phospholipids, is extremely valuable in case of increase in cholesterol level. It has the ability to break up cholesterol into small particles which can be effortlessly handled by the system. With adequate intake of lecithin, cholesterol cannot build up against the walls of the arteries and veins. It also increases the production of bile acids made from cholesterol, thus reducing its amount in the blood.

Vegetable oils, whole grain cereals, egg yolk, soyabeans and unpasteurised milk are rich sources of lecithin. The cells of the body are also competent of synthesising it as needed, if several of the B vitamins are present. Diets high in vitamin B6, cholin and inositol supplied by wheat germ, yeast, or B vitamins extracted from bran have been predominantly successful in reducing blood cholesterol. Sometimes vitamin E elevates blood lecithin and reduces cholesterol presumably by preventing the necessary fatty acids from being destroyed by oxygen. Persons with high blood cholesterol level should drink at least eight to ten glasses of water every day as regular drinking of water stimulates the excretory activity of the skin and kidneys. This in turn facilitates elimination of excessive cholesterol from the system. Drinking of coriander (dhania) water on a regular basis also helps lower blood cholesterol as it is a good diuretic and stimulates the kidneys. It is prepared by boiling dry seeds of coriander and straining the decoction after cooling.

Regular exercise also plays a significant part in lowering LDL cholesterol and in raising the level of protective high density lipoproteins (HDL). It also promotes circulation and helps maintain the blood flow to every part of the body. Jogging or brisk walking, swimming, bicycling and playing badminton are excellent forms of exercise. Yoga asanas are greatly favourable as they help increase perspiratory activity and stimulate sebaceous glands to effectively secrete accumulated or excess cholesterol from the muscular tissue. Asanas like ardha matsyaendrasana, salabhasana, padmasana and vajrasana are useful in lowering blood cholesterol by increasing systemic activity. Hydrotherapy can be effectively employed in reducing surplus cholesterol. Cold hip baths for ten minutes taken twice every day have proved beneficial. Steam baths are also helpful apart from patients suffering from hypertension and other circulatory disorders. Mud packs, applied over the abdomen improve digestion and assimilation. They improve the functioning of the liver and other digestive organs and activate kidneys and the intestines to encourage better excretion.

Chapter 28

Habitual Abortion

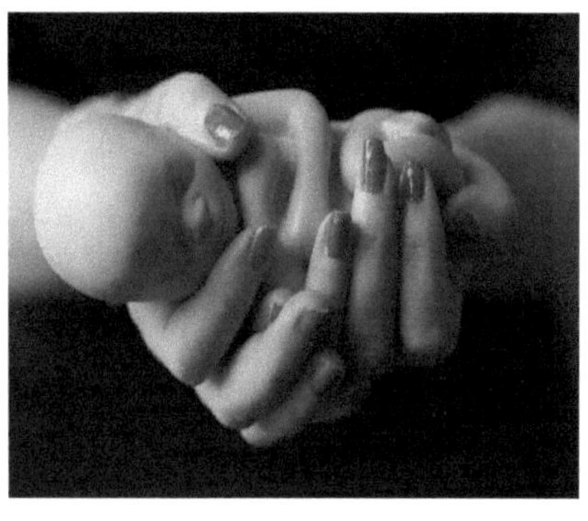

In the natural remedy for habitual abortion the patient should be put to bed immediately and the bottom end of the bed raised on appearance of the first symptoms of possible abortion. Cold compresses at 60 degrees Fahrenheit temperatures should be applied constantly to the inner portion of the thighs, the vagina and the lumbar region. Compresses should be changed every fifteen to twenty minutes. When the compress is removed for renewing, the surface should be rubbed with a warm dry flannel for half a minute or until reddened, before applying the compress again. At the same time, a hot application should be made to the feet.

A neutral or lukewarm water enema is a useful remedy for a constipated colon which is a major reason for the toxaemic condition of the uterus. This will ease the bowels and thus lessen any excessive pressure on the uterus and other pelvic organs. A regular cold hip bath for duration of ten minutes twice every day is very useful in relieving congestion and inflammation of the uterus. Wet girdle packs, twice every day, on an empty stomach, also relieve congestion's and infections in the uterus and other pelvic organs. It is wise that women with a history of repeated abortions should take on these techniques before conception and maintain them during the first two months of pregnancy.

Hormonal imbalances can be set right by practicing yogic exercise. Yoga asanas such as sarvangasana, vajrasana, bhujangasana, salabhsana, dhanurasana, paschimottashana, and trikonasana are particularly helpful in improving thyroid, pituitary, and adrenal and gonaidal endocrine functions and should be practiced on a regular basis by women who suffer from imbalances of this sort, up to the first two months of pregnancy. Dietary control is of supreme importance in the prevention of habitual abortion. Pregnant women should avoid refined carbohydrates, non vegetarian food, coffee, sugars, and tea. They should also keep away from oily and fried foods as such foods lead to constipation, which is very harmful to pregnancy. Smoking or chewing tobacco and drinking alcohol must be strictly avoided.

The pregnant woman's diet chart should be on the following lines:

- **Breakfast:** Fresh fruits and a glass of milk mixed with a teaspoonful of honey.
- **Lunch:** Steamed vegetables, boiled rice or whole wheat chappatis and soup or buttermilk.
- **Mid afternoon:** A glass of fruit juice or a whole fruit.
- **Dinner:** Cooked diet similar to the afternoon meal may be taken till the seventh month. After that, fruits, nuts, milk, buttermilk and soups, germinated seeds and sprouts, must form her diet because they decrease the workload on the digestive system and thus help avoid indigestion, constipation and related disorders.

Indian gooseberry, known as amla in the Hindi, is considered useful in preventing abortion. A teaspoonful of fresh amla juice and honey mixed together should be taken every morning during the period of pregnancy. It will also prevent infections and assist in the absorption of iron. A brew made from safflower foliage is also said to avert abortion. Pregnant women with a history of repeated abortions should take all other precautions essential to prevent miscarriage. They should stay away from sexual intercourse, during early pregnancy. They should go to bed early and rise early and take regular exercise, but avoid fatigue. They should sleep on a hard mattress with their heads low, and remain calm and cool. All these measures will to a great extent help in correcting the phenomenon of habitual abortion.

Chapter 29

Bronchitis

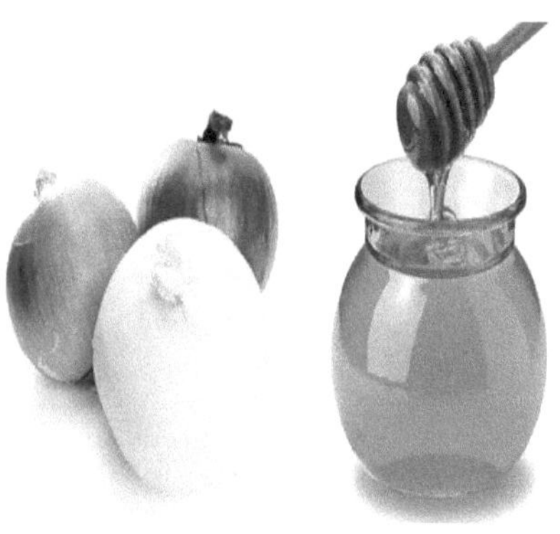

In the natural remedy for bronchitis it is advisable that the patient should fast on orange juice and water till the severe symptoms fall down. The procedure is to take the juice of an orange in a glass of warm water every two hours from 8 a.m. to 8 p.m. After that, the patient should take up an all-fruit diet for two or three days. In case of chronic bronchitis, the patient should begin with an all- fruit diet for five to seven days, taking each day three meals of fresh juicy fruits. After the all-fruit diet, the patient should follow a well-balanced diet of seeds, nuts and grains, vegetables and fruits. For drinks, unsweetened lemon water or cold or hot plain water may be taken. The patient should keep away from meats, sugar, tea, coffee, condiments, pickles, refined and processed foods, soft-drinks, candies, ice-cream and products made from sugar and white flour.

One of the most successful medications for bronchitis is the use of turmeric powder. A teaspoonful of this powder should be administered with a glass of milk two or three times daily. It acts best when taken on an empty stomach. Another effective cure for bronchitis is a mixture of dried ginger powder, pepper and long pepper taken in the same quantities three times a day. It may be licked with honey or infused with one's daily tea. The powder of these three ingredients has antipyretic qualities and is effective in dealing with fever accompanied by bronchitis. They also tone up the metabolism of the patient.

The onion has been used as a food remedy for centuries in bronchitis. It is said to possess expectorant properties. It liquefies phelgm and prevents its additional formation.

A hot Epsom-salts bath every night or every other night will be extremely helpful during the acute stages of the attack. This bath is prepared by dissolving three table spoons of Epsom-salts to sixty litres of water having a temperature of 100 degree F. The patient should stay immersed in the bath for about twenty minutes. In case of chronic bronchitis, this bath may be taken twice a week. Hot towels wrung out and applied over the upper chest are also helpful. After applying three hot towels in turn for two or three minutes each, one should always finish off with a cold towel. A cold pack should also be applied to the upper chest quite a few times daily in acute conditions. The procedure is to wring out some linen material in cold water, wrap two or three times round the affected part and cover it with some flannel. The pack can remain for about an hour at a time.

Fresh air and outdoor exercises are also indispensable to the treatment of bronchitis and the patient should take a good walk everyday. He should also perform yogic kriyas such as jalaneti and vamandhouti and yogic asanas such as ekpaduttansana, yogamudra, bhujangasana, salabhasana, padmasana and shavasana. Simple pranayama like kapalbhati, anuloma-viloma, ujjai and bhramari are also highly beneficial.

Chapter 30

Cirrhosis of Liver

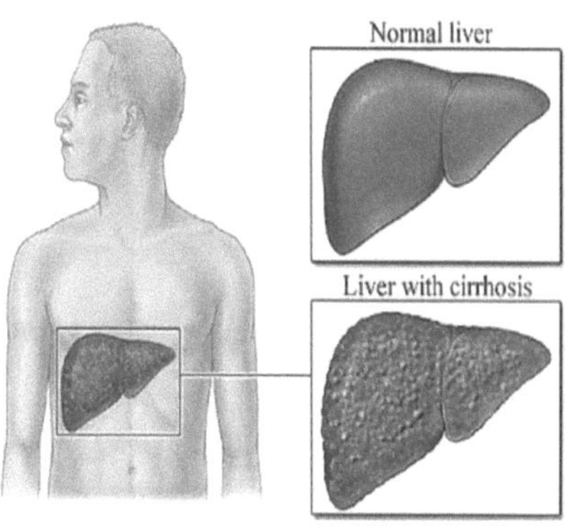

Naturopathy offers a natural remedy for cirrhosis of liver. The patient should be given complete bed rest and must abstain from alcohol in any form. Initially the patient should undergo an initial liver cleaning programme with a juice fast for seven days. Freshly extracted juices from red beets, lemon, papaya and grapes may be taken all through this period. This may be followed by the fruit and milk diet for two to three weeks. In this regimen, the patient should have three meals a day, each of fresh juicy fruits and milk.

The fruits may include apples, pears, grapes, grape fruit, pineapples and peaches. One litre of milk may be taken on the first day. It should be increased by 250 ml. daily up to two to two and a half litres a day. The milk should be fresh and may be slightly warmed if desired.

Following the fruit and milk diet, the patient may gradually embark upon a well-balanced diet of three basic food groups, namely (i) seeds, nuts and grains, (ii) vegetables and (iii) fruits, with emphasis on raw organically grown foods. A sufficient high quality protein diet is necessary in cirrhosis. The best complete proteins for liver patients are obtained from raw goat`s milk, home-made raw cottage cheese, sprouted seeds and grains and raw nuts, especially almonds. Vegetables such as beets, squashes, bitter gourd, egg-plant, tomato, carrot, radishes and papaya are helpful in this condition. All fats and oils should be excluded from the diet for several weeks.

The patient should avoid all refined, processed and canned foods, sugar in any form, spices and condiments, strong tea and coffee, fried foods, all preparations cooked in ghee, oil or butter and all meats rich in fat. The use of salt should be constrained. The patient should also keep away from all chemical additives in food and poisons in air, water and environment. Warm water enema should be used during the treatment to cleanse the bowels. If constipation is habitual, all steps should be taken for its eradication. Application of alternate compress to liver area followed by general wet sheet rub is useful. The morning dry friction and breathing and other exercises should form a regular daily aspect of the treatment.

Chapter 31

Constipation

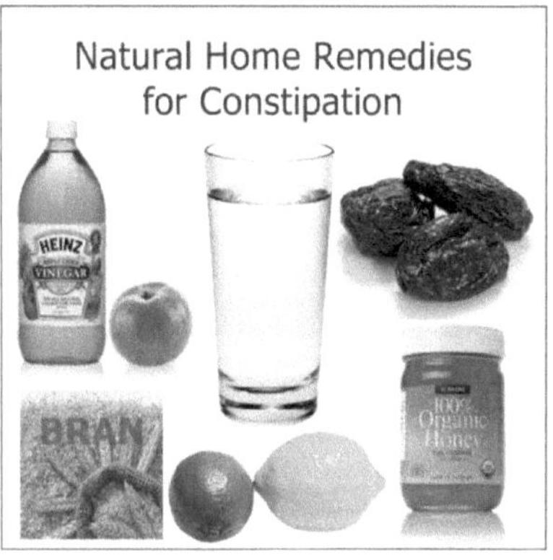

Diet is the most significant factor in the natural cure of constipation. This should consist of unrefined food such as whole grain cereals, honey, molasses, and lentils; green and leafy vegetables, especially spinach, tomatoes, lettuce, onion, cabbage, cauliflower, sprouts, celery, turnip, pumpkin, peas, beets, asparagus and carrot. Fresh fruits, particularly pears, grapes, figs, papayas, mangoes, grapefruit, gooseberries, guava and oranges; dry fruits such as figs, raisins, apricots and dates; milk products in the form of butter, ghee and cream are to be included in the diet.

The diet alone is not enough. Food should be properly chewed-each morsel for at least fifteen times. Hurried meals and meals at odd times should be avoided. Sugar and sugary foods should be firmly avoided because sugar steals B vitamins from the body, without which the intestines cannot function normally. Regular drinking of water is beneficial not only for constipation but also for cleaning the system, diluting the blood and washing out poisons. Normally six to eight glasses of water should be taken every day as it is necessary for digesting and dissolving food nutrients so that they can be absorbed and utilised by the body. Water should, however, not be taken with meals as it dilutes the gastric juices essential for proper digestion. Water should be taken either half an hour before or an hour after meals.

Generally all fruits, except banana and jack fruit are beneficial in the treatment of constipation. Certain fruits are however, more effective. Bael fruit is regarded as best of all laxatives. It cleans and tones up the intestines. Its normal use for two or three months throws out even the old accumulated faucal matter. Though generally used to check diarrhoea, bael contains both laxative and constipative properties. It hardens the stools when they are loose and serves as a laxative when the bowels are constipated. Pears are regarded the next best fruit useful in the treatment of constipation. Patients suffering from chronic constipation should better adopt an exclusive diet of this fruit or its juice for few days, but in normal cases a medium-sized pear taken after dinner or with breakfast will have the desired result. The same is true of guava which, when eaten with seeds, gives roughage to the diet and helps in the normal evacuation of the bowels.

Grapes have also proved extremely beneficial in overcoming constipation. The combination of the properties of the cellulose, sugar and organic acid in grapes make them a laxative food. Their field of action is not limited to clearing the bowels only. They also tone up the stomach and intestines and relieve the most chronic constipation. One should take at least 350 grams of grapes daily to achieve the desired results. When fresh grapes are not available, raisins soaked in water can be used. Raisins should be soaked in drinking water for 24 to 48 hours. This would swell them to the original size of the grapes. The raisins should be eaten early in the morning. The water in which raisins are soaked should be drunk along with the soaked raisins.

Drinking hot water with sour lime juice and half a teaspoon of salt is also an effective remedy for constipation. Linseed is very useful in difficult cases of constipation. A teaspoon of linseed swallowed with water before each meal provides both bulk and lubrication. In all ordinary cases of constipation, an exclusive fruit diet for about seven days would be the best way to begin the treatment. Weak patients may take orange juice during the period of fasting. After the all-fruit diet or the short fast, as the case may be, the patient should gradually embark upon a balanced diet comprising adequate raw foods, ripe fruits and whole grain cereals. It some cases, further short periods on fruits or short fasts may be essential at intervals of two months or so, depending on the improvement being made. The bowels should be cleansed daily through a warm water enema for a few days at the commencement of the treatment.

A cold friction bath taken daily in the morning can help cure constipation. An alternate hot and cold hit bath taken before retiring to bed is also beneficial. Abdominal exercise and manual or mechanical vibratory massage have a refreshing and stimulating effect in many cases. Toning up the muscles also helps in the treatment of constipation.

Fresh air, outdoor games, walking, swimming, gardening and exercise play an important role in strengthening and activating the muscles, thereby preventing constipation. Yoga for constipation brings relief as they strengthen the abdominal and pelvic muscles and stimulate the peristalic action of the bowels. These asanas are: bhujansana, salabhasana, yogamudra, dhanurasana, halasana, paschimottanasana. Pranayamas, such as, anuloma-viloma and bhastrika and jalaneti kriyas are also helpful.

Chapter 32

Appendicitis

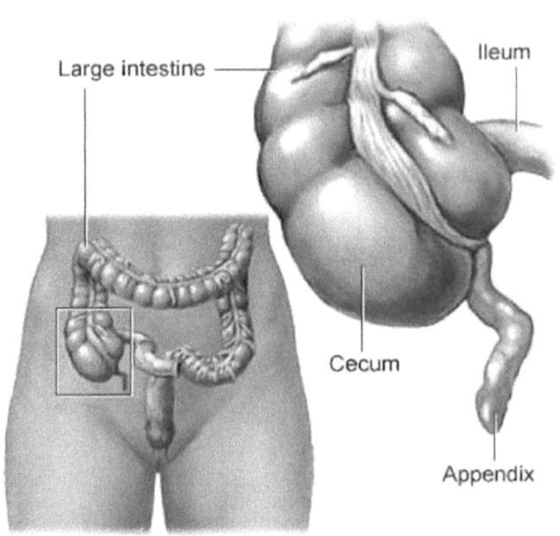

Natural Remedy for Appendicitis in Indian Naturopathy is rest and fasting. Rest is of utmost importance in the treatment of this disease. The patient should resort to fasting which is the only real therapy for appendicitis. Absolutely no food should be given. Nothing except water should enter the body. Low enemas, containing about one pint (1/2 litre) of warm water should be administered everyday for the first three days to cleanse the lower bowel. Hot compresses may be placed over the painful area a number of times daily. Abdominal packs, made of a strip of wet sheet covered by a dry flannel cloth bound tightly around the abdomen, should be applied constantly until all acute symptoms settles.

After the acute symptoms subside by about the third day, the patient should be given a full enema containing about one and half litre of warm water and this should be repeated daily until the inflammation and pain have subsided. The patient can be given fruit juices from the third day onwards. This simple treatment wisely applied will overcome an appendicitis attack. After spending three days on fruit juices, the patient may adopt an all-fruit diet for further four or five days. During this period, he should have three meals a day each meal of fresh juicy fruits. Thereafter, he should adopt a well-balanced diet based on three food groups namely, (i) seed, nuts and grains, (ii) vegetables and (iii) fruits.

In case of chronic appendicitis, a short fast should be followed by a full milk diet for two or three weeks. In this routine, a glass of milk should be taken every two hours from 8 a.m. to 8 p.m. on the first day, a glass every hour and a half the next day and a glass every hour the third day. Then the quantity of milk should be gradually increased so as to take a glass every half an hour, if such a quantity can be tolerated comfortably. After the full milk diet, the patient should gradually embark upon a well- balanced diet, with emphasis on fresh fruits and green leafy vegetables.

Certain vegetable juices, especially carrot juice, in combination with the juices of beets and cucumbers, have been found helpful in the treatment of appendicitis. Regular use of tea made from fenugreek seeds has also proved helpful in preventing the appendix from becoming a dumping ground for excess mucous and intestinal waste. The patient of appendicitis should adopt all measures to eliminate constipation, if it is habitual. Much relief can be obtained by the application of hot fomentation and abdominal packs every morning and night. An abdominal massage is also advantageous. Once the waste matter in the calcium has moved into the colon and thence eliminated, the irritation and inflammation in the appendix will subside and surgical removal of the appendix will not be required. The surgical operation should be resorted to only in rare cases, when the appendix has become abscessed.

Chapter 33

Asthma

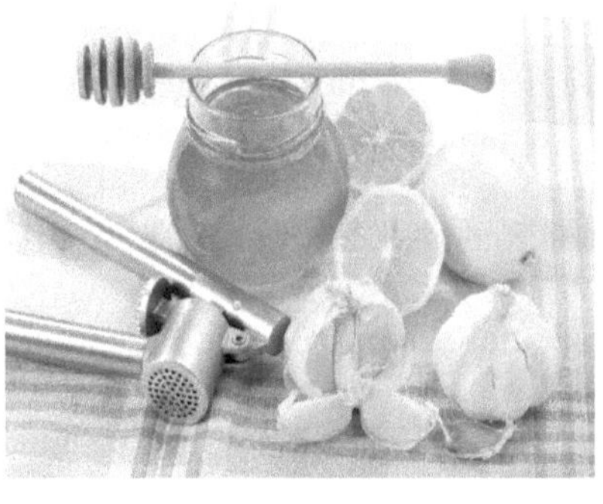

Natural way to treat asthma involves stimulating the functioning of relaxed excretory organs, adopting proper diet patterns to remove morbid matter and renovate the body. Practicing yoga asanas, yogic kriyas and Pranayama is also necessary to allow proper assimilation of food and to strengthen the lungs, digestive system and circulatory organs. The patient should be given an enema to clean the colon and prevent auto-intoxication.

Mud-packs applied to the abdomen will ease the fermentation caused by undigested food and will promote intestinal peristalsis. Wet packs should be applied to the chest to lessen the congestion of the lungs and strengthen them. The patient should be made to perspire through steam bath, hot foot bath, hot hip bath and sun bath. This will stimulate the skin and relieve congested lungs.

The patient should fast for a few days on lemon juice with honey and thereafter resort to a fruit juice diet to nurture the system and remove the toxins. Gradually, solid foods can be included in the diet. Ideally diet should contain a limited quantity of carbohydrates, fats and proteins which are acid-forming foods, and a liberal quantity of alkaline foods consisting of fresh fruits, green vegetables and germinated gram. Foods which tend to produce phelgm such as rice, sugar, lentils and curds as also fried and other difficult- to- digest foods should be avoided. Breakfast may consist of prunes, orange or berries or a few black raisins with honey. Lunch and dinner should consist of a salad of raw vegetables such as cucumber, lettuce, tomato, carrot and beets, one or two lightly cooked green vegetables and wheat bread.

Asthmatics should always eat less than their capacity. They should eat slowly, chewing their food properly. They should drink eight to ten glasses of water a day, but should avoid taking water or any liquid with meals. Spices, chillies and pickles, too much tea and coffee should also be avoided. Asthma, particularly when the attack is severe, tends to destroy the appetite. In such cases, the patient should be kept on fast till the attack is over. Honey is considered highly advantageous in the treatment of asthma. Honey usually brings respite whether the air flowing over it is inhaled or whether it is eaten or taken either in milk or water. Another successful remedy for asthma is garlic. Turmeric is also regarded as an effective remedy for bronchial asthma. The patient should be given a teaspoonful of turmeric powder with a glass of milk two or three times on a daily basis.

During the attack, mustard oil mixed with little camphor should be massaged over the back of the chest. This will loosen up phelgm and ease breathing. The patient should also inhale steam from the boiling water with caraway seeds, known as ajwain in the vernacular. It will dilate the bronchial passage. The patient should also follow the other laws of nature. Regular fasting once a week, an occasional enema, breathing exercises, fresh air, dry climate, light exercises and a correct posture go a long way in treating the disease. The patient should perform yogic kriyas such as jalneti, vamandhouti and yogic asanas such as ekpaduttanasana, yogamudra, sarvangasana, padmasana, bhujangasana, dhanurasana, vakrasana, ardha matsyendrasana, salabhasan, paschimottanasana and shavasana. Pranayamas like kapalbhati, anuloma-viloma, ujjayi, suryabhedana and bhramari are also highly beneficial.

Chapter 34

Dandruff

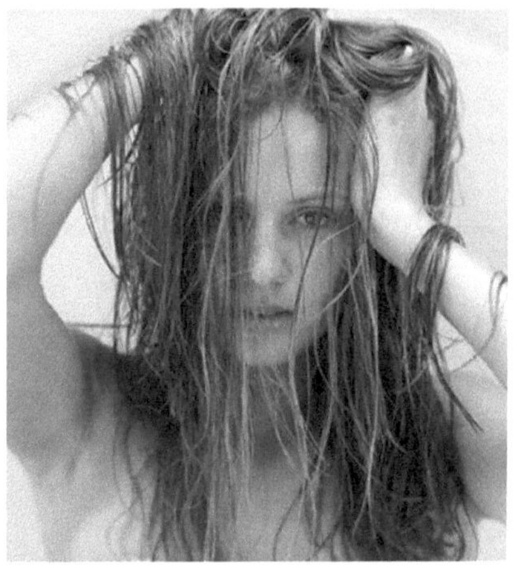

Natural remedy of dandruff prescribes the cleansing of the hair and scalp. Proper cleaning of hair and the scalp will minimise the growth of dead cells. The hair should be brushed daily to improve the circulation and remove any flakiness. The most successful way to brush the hair is to bend forward from the waist with the head down towards the ground, and brush from the nape of the neck towards the top of the head. Short or shoulder length hair can be brushed right from the roots to the ends in one stroke. In the case of long hair, two strokes would be best to avoid stretching the hair. The scalp should also be thoroughly massaged every day, using one's finger tips and working systematically over the head. This should be done just before or after brushing the hair. Like brushing, this stimulates the circulation, dislodges dirt and dandruff and encourages hair growth.

A proper massage helps in the removal of dandruff. A number of home remedies have been found useful in the treatment of dandruff. The use of fenugreek (methi) seeds is one such remedy. Two tablespoons of fenugreek seeds should be soaked overnight in water. The softer seeds should be ground into a fine paste in the morning. This paste should be applied all over the scalp and left for half-an hour. The hair should then be washed thoroughly with soap nut (ritha) solution or shikakai. The use of a teaspoon of fresh lime juice for the last rinse, while washing hair, is equally useful. This not only leaves the hair glowing but also removes stickiness and prevents dandruff. Washing the hair twice a week with green gram powder in curd is another useful recommendation.

Dandruff can be removed by massaging one's hair or half-an- hour with curd which has been kept in the open for three days, or with a few drops of lime juice mixed with amla juice every night, before going to bed. Another measure which helps to thwart dandruff is to dilute cider vinegar with an equal quantity of water and dab this on to the hair with cotton wool in between shampooing. Cider vinegar added to the final rinsing water after shampooing also helps to disperse dandruff. Diet plays an imperative role in the treatment of dandruff. To begin with, the patient should resort to all fruit diet for about five days. In this regimen, there should be three meals a day, consisting of fresh, juicy fruits, such as apples, pears, grapes, grapefruit, pineapple and peaches. Citrus fruits, bananas, dried, strewed or tinned fruits should not be taken. Only unsweetened lemon or plain water, either hot or cold, should be drunk. During this period, a warm water enema should be taken on a daily basis to cleanse the bowels and all other measures adopted to eradicate constipation.

After the all fruit diet, the patient can steadily adopt a well balanced diet. Emphasis should be on raw foods, chiefly fresh fruits and vegetables; sprouted seeds, raw nuts and whole grain cereals, particularly millet and brown rice. Further short periods on the all-fruits diet for three days or so may be required at a monthly interval, till the skin's condition improves. Strict attention to diet is essential for resurgence. Starchy, protein, and fatty foods should be restricted. Meats, sugar, strong tea or coffee, condiments, pickles, refined and processed foods all these should be avoided, as also soft drinks, candies, ice cream and products made with sugar and white flour. Exposure of the head to the rays of the sun is also a functional measure in the treatment of dandruff. At the same time, an attempt should be made to keep the body in good health. This also helps clear dandruff.

Chapter 35

Diabetes

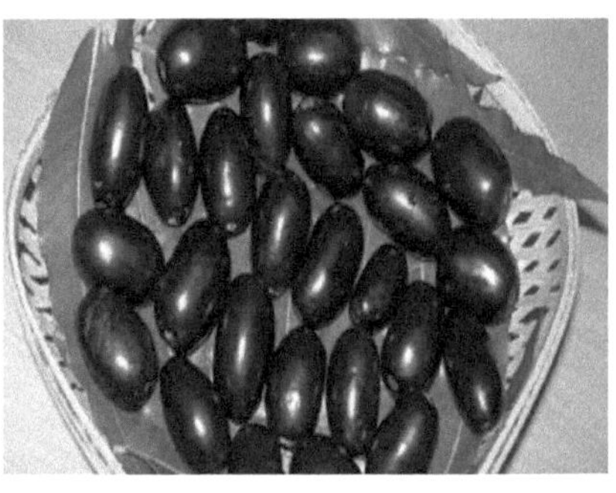

Natural remedy of diabetes involves the removal of the actual cause of the disease with the help of a proper and balanced diet. The primary dietary consideration for a diabetic patient is that he should be a strict lacto-vegetarian and take a low-calorie, low-fat, alkaline diet of high quality natural foods. Fruits, nuts and vegetables, whole meal bread and dairy products form a good diet for the diabetic. These foods are best eaten in as dry a condition as possible to guarantee thorough salivation during the first part of the process of digestion. Cooked starchy foods should be avoided as in the process of cooking the cellulose envelops of the starch granules burst and consequently, the starch is far too easily absorbed in the system. The excess absorbed has to be got rid of by the kidneys and appears as sugar in the urine.

The diabetic should eat fresh fruits and vegetables which contain sugar and starch. Fresh fruits contain sugar fructose, which does not need insulin for its metabolism and is well tolerated by diabetics. Emphasis should be on raw foods as they stimulate and increase insulin production. For protein, home- made cottage cheese, various forms of soured milks and nuts are best. The patient should avoid overeating and take four or five small meals a day rather than three large ones.

The following diet should serve as a guideline:

- **Breakfast:** Any fresh fruit with the exception of bananas, soaked prunes a small quantity of whole meal bread with butter and fresh milk.
- **Lunch:** Steamed or lightly cooked green vegetables such as cauliflower, cabbage, tomatoes, spinach, turnip, asparagus and

mushrooms, two or three whole wheat chapatis according to appetite and a glass of butter-milk or curd.

- **Mid-afternoon:** A glass of fresh fruit or vegetable juice.
- **Dinner:** A large bowl of salad made up of all the raw vegetables in season. The salad may be followed by a hot course, if desired, and fresh home-made cottage cheese.
- **Bedtime Snack:** A glass of fresh milk.

Flesh foods find no place in this regimen, for they increase the toxaemic state underlying the diabetic state and lessen the sugar tolerance. On the other hand, a non-stimulating vegetarian diet, in particular one made up of raw foods, promotes and increases sugar tolerance. Celery, cucumbers, string beans, onion and garlic are especially advantageous. String bean pod tea is an excellent natural replacement for insulin and highly useful in diabetes. The skin of the pods of green beans is very rich in silica and certain hormone substances which are strongly related to insulin. One cup of string bean tea is equal to one unit of insulin. Cucumbers contain a hormone needed by the cells of the pancreas for producing insulin. Onion and garlic have proved beneficial in reducing blood sugar in diabetes.

Recent scientific investigations have established that bitter gourd or karela is extremely beneficial in the treatment of diabetes. It contains an insulin-like principle, known as plant-insulin which has been found effectual in lowering the blood and urine sugar levels. It should, therefore, be included abundantly in the diet of the diabetic. For better results, the diabetic should take the juice of about four or five fruits every morning on an empty stomach. The seeds of bitter gourd can be added to food in a powdered form. Diabetics can also use bitter gourd in the form of decoction by boiling the pieces in water or in the form of dry powder. Another effective home medication is jambul fruit known as jamun in the vernacular. It is regarded in traditional medicine as a specific against diabetes because of its effect on the pancreas.

The seeds of the fruits and fruit juice are all useful in the treatment of this disease. The seeds contain a glucoside `jamboline` which is believed to have power to check the pathological conversion of starch into sugar in cases of increased production of glucose. The patient should avoid tea, coffee and cocoa because of their adverse influence on the digestive tract. Other foods which should be avoided are white bread, white flour products, sugar tinned fruits, sweets, chocolates, pastries, pies, puddings, refined cereals and alcoholic drinks. The most important nutrient in the treatment of diabetes is manganese which is very important in the production of natural insulin. It is found in citrus fruits, in the outer covering of nuts, grains and in the green leaves of edible plants. Other nutrients of special value are zinc, B complex vitamins and poly-unsaturated fatty acids.

Exercise is also an inseparable factor in the treatment of diabetes. Light games, jogging and swimming are recommended. Yogic asanas such as bhujangasana, salabhasana, dhanurasana, paschimottanasana, sarvangasna, halasana, ardha-matsyendrasana and shavasana, yogic kriyas like jalneti and kunaji and pranayamas such as kapalbhati, anuloma-viloma and ujjai are very much beneficial. Hydrotherapy and colonic irrigations form a very imperative part of treatment. The colon should be methodically cleansed every second day or so, until the bowel discharge assumes normal characteristics. Bathing in cold water significantly increases the circulation and enhances the ability of the muscles to utilise sugar. The diabetic patient should eliminate minor worries from his daily life. He or she must endeavour to be more easy-going and should not get excessively worked up by the stress and strain of life.

Chapter 36

Eczema

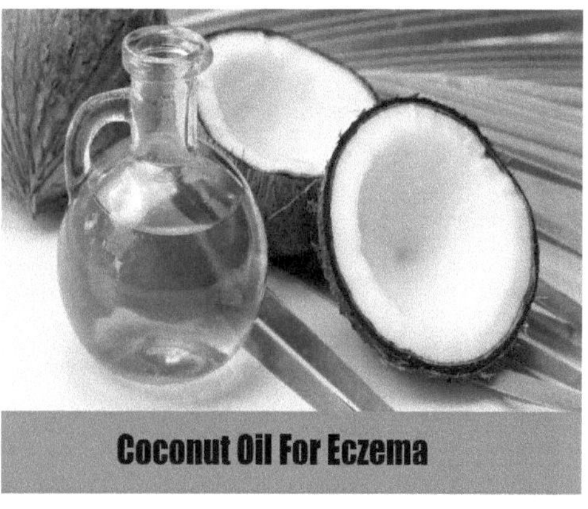

Coconut Oil For Eczema

Natural remedy for eczema should start with a fast on orange juice and water from five to days, depending on the severity and duration of the trouble. Juice fasting, helps to eliminate toxic waste from the body and leads to considerable development. In some cases, the condition may deteriorate in the beginning of the fast due to the increased exclusion of waste matter through the skin. But as fasting continues, improvement will manifest itself. Fruits, salt free, raw or steamed vegetables with whole meal bread or chappatis may be taken after the juice fast. Carrot and musk melon are chiefly beneficial. Coconut oil may be used instead of ghee. After a few days, curd and milk may be added to the diet. The patients may after that, gradually embark upon a well-balanced diet of three basic food groups, namely (i) seeds, nuts and grains (ii) vegetables and (iii) fruits.

Huge proportion of the diet should comprise raw foods. Seeds and beans such as alfalfa and soyabeans can be sprouted. This diet may be supplemented with cold-pressed vegetable oils, honey and yeast. Juice fasting may be repeated at intervals of two months or so, depending on the improvement being made, in chronic and more difficult cases of eczema, patient should fast at least once a week till he is cured. The patient should avoid tea, coffee, alcoholic beverages and all condiments and highly flavoured dishes. He should also avoid sugar, white flour products, denatured cereals like polished rice, and pearled barley and tinned or bottled foods. He should eat only unadulterated and wholesome foods. Raw vegetable juices, particularly carrot juice in combination with spinach juice, have proved highly advantageous in the treatment of eczema.

Fresh air is advisable for the patient. Restrictive clothing should not be worn. Two or three liters of water should be taken on a daily basis and the patient must bath twice or thrice a day. The skin, with the exception of the parts affected with eczema, should be vigorously rubbed with the palms of the hands before taking the bath. Coconut oil may be applied to the portions with eczema. It will help the skin to stay soft. Walking or jogging should be resorted to in order to inactivate the bowels. Sun bathing is also favourable as it kills the harmful bacteria and should be resorted to early in the morning, in the first light of dawn. A light mudpack should be applied over the sites of the eczema is also helpful. The pack should be applied for an hour at a time and should be repeated twice or thrice a day.

In cases of acute eczema, cold compress or cold wet fomentations are beneficial. The affected part should be wrapped with a thick soft cloth. The cloth should be moistened with cold water (55 degrees Fahrenheit to 60 degrees Fahrenheit) every fifteen to thirty minutes for two hours at a time. The bandage should be left intact, keeping the cloth cold. There may be intensification of itching or pain in the beginning but it will soon subside. A cold compress may be applied twice daily for a week or so.

Chapter 37

Gastritis

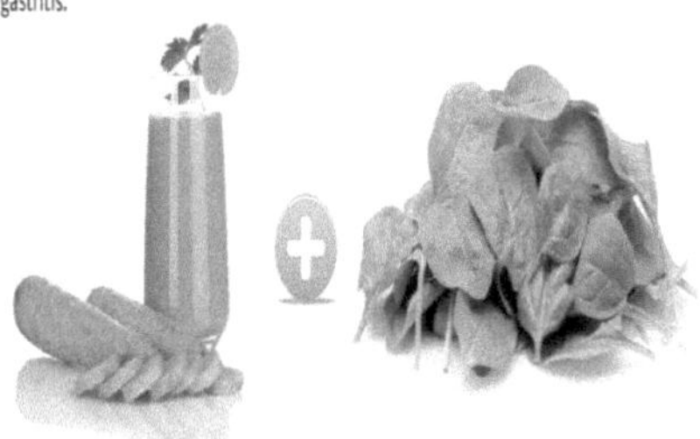
Mix half cup of carrot juice and equal amount of spinach juice and drink for chronic gastritis.

In Naturopathy, the natural remedy for gastritis is to take on a fast in both acute and chronic cases. In acute cases, the patient will usually recover after a short fast of two or three days. In chronic condition, the fast may have to be continued for a longer period of seven days or so. The fast may be conducted on fruit juices. By fasting, the intake of irritants is at once successfully stopped, the stomach is rested and the toxic condition, causing the inflammation, is allowed to settle. After the acute symptoms subside, the patient should adopt an all-fruit diet for further three days. Juicy fruits such as apple, pear, grapes, orange, pineapple, peach and melon may be taken during this period at five-hourly intervals.

The patient can after that gradually embarks upon a well balanced diet of three basic food groups, namely: (i) seeds, nuts and grains, (ii) vegetables, and (iii) fruits on the following lines:

- **Breakfast:** Fresh fruits, such as apples, orange, banana, grapes, grapefruit or any available berries, a handful of raw nuts and a glass of milk.
- **Mid-morning snack:** One apple, banana, or any other fruit.
- **Lunch:** Steamed vegetables, two or three slices of whole meal bread or whole wheat chappatis, according to the appetite and a glass of butter milk.
- **Mid-afternoon:** A glass of fresh fruit or vegetable juice or sugarcane juice.
- **Dinner:** A large bowl of fresh salad of green vegetables such as tomatoes, carrots, red beets, cabbage, and cucumber with dressing of lemon juice and cold-pressed vegetable oil, all accessible sprouts such as alfalfa seeds, fresh butter and fresh

home made cottage cheese. Bed time snacks: A glass of fresh milk or one apple.

The use of alcohol, nicotine, spices, and condiments, flesh foods, chilies, sour things, pickles, strong tea and coffee should be avoided by the patient. He should also avoid sweets, pastries, cakes and aerated waters. Carrot juice in combination with the juice of spinach is considered highly advantageous in the treatment of gastritis. Too many different foods should not be mixed at the same meal. Meals should be taken at least two hours before going to bed at night. Eight to ten glasses of water should be taken on a daily basis but water should not be taken with meals as it dilutes the digestive juices and delays digestion. And above all, haste should be avoided while eating and meals should be served in a pleasant and relaxed atmosphere.

Coconut water is an excellent food remedy for gastritis. It gives the stomach needed rest and provides vitamins and minerals. The stomach will be significantly helped in returning to its normal condition if nothing except coconut water is given during the first twenty four hours. Rice gruel is another effective medication in acute cases of gastritis. In chronic cases where the flow of gastric juice is meagre, such foods as require prolonged vigorous mastication will be beneficial as this induces a greater flow of gastric juices. From the beginning of the treatment, a warm water enema should be used on a daily basis, for about a week, to cleanse the bowels. If constipation is habitual, all steps should be taken for its eradication.

The patient should be given daily a dry friction and sponge bath. Application of heat, through hot compressor or hot water bottle twice in the day either on an empty stomach or two hours after meals, should also prove beneficial. The patient should not undertake any hard physical and mental work. He should, however, undertake breathing and other light exercises like walking, swimming, and golf. He should avoid worries and mental tension.

Chapter 38

Gout

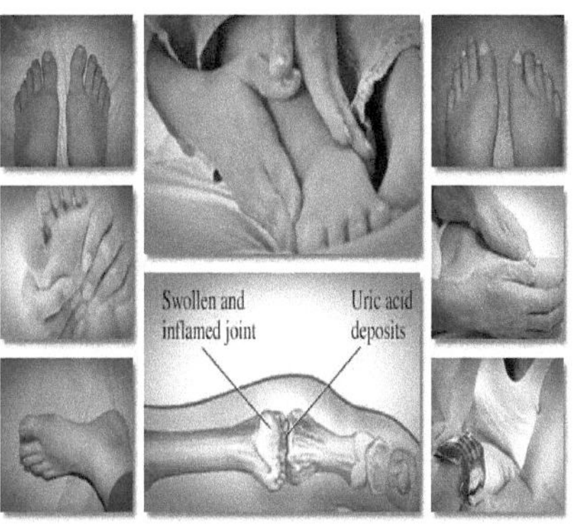

In Naturopathy, there is no better natural remedy than a fast for the treatment of Gout. The patient should embark on a fast for five to seven days on orange juice and water. In severe cases, it is advisable to undertake a series of short fasts for three days or so rather than one long fast. Warm water enema should be used on a daily basis during the period of fasting to cleanse the bowels. After the acute symptoms of gout have subsided, the patient may adopt an all-fruit diet for further three or four days. In this regimen, he should have three meals a day of juicy fruits such as grapes, apples, pears, peaches, oranges and pineapple.

After the all-fruit diet, the patient may slowly embark upon the following diet:

- **Breakfast:** Fruits such as oranges, apples, figs, apricot, mangoes, whole wheat bread or dalia and milk or butter-milk.
- **Lunch:** Steamed vegetables such as lettuce, beets, celery, water-cress, turnips, squash, carrots, tomatoes, cabbage and potatoes, chappatis of whole wheat flour, cottage cheese and butter-milk.
- **Dinner:** Sprouts such as alfalfa, a good-sized salad of raw vegetables such as carrots, cabbage, tomatoes, whole wheat bread and butter.

The patient should avoid uric acid producing foods such as all meats, eggs, and fish. Glandular meats are in particular harmful. He should also avoid all intoxicating liquors, tea, coffee, sugar, white flour and its products and all canned and processed foods. Spices and salts should be used as little as possible. The cherry, sweet or sour, is considered a successful medication for gout. To start with, the patient should consume about fifteen to twenty five cherries a day. Thereafter, about ten cherries a day will keep the disease under control. Foods high in potassium such as potatoes, bananas, leafy green vegetables, beans and raw vegetable juices are protective against gout. Carrot juice in combination with juices of beet and cucumber is particularly valuable.

The juice of french or string beans has also proved effective in the healing of gout. Raw potato juice and fresh pineapple juices are also beneficial. The feet should be bathed in Epsom salt foot bath twice on a daily basis. Half a pound to one pound of salt may be added to a foot bath of hot water. Full Epsom salt baths should also be taken three times a week. The baths may be reduced to two per week later. Cold packs at night, applied to the affected joints, will be advantageous. Fresh air and outdoor exercise are also indispensable. The patient should get rid of as much stress from his life as possible.

Chapter 39

Hydrocele

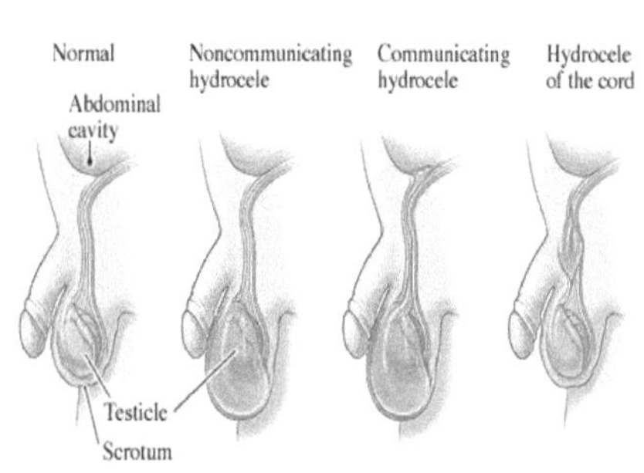

In the natural remedy for hydrocele, the sufferer should begin with an exclusive fresh fruit diet for seven to ten days. In this regimen, he should have three meals a day of fresh juicy fruits, such as apples, pears, grapes, grape fruit, oranges, pineapple, peaches, melon or any other juicy fruit in season. For drinks, lemon water unsweetened or water either hot or cold may be taken. During this period the bowels should be cleansed on a daily basis with a warm water enema. If constipation is habitual, all steps should be taken for its eradication.

After all all-fruit diet the patient may adopt the following regimen:

- **Breakfast:** Fresh fruit as obtainable, or grated raw carrot or other raw salad stuff, prunes or other dried fruits, if desired, and a cup of milk.
- **Lunch:** Steamed vegetables, as obtainable, with either a poached or scrambled egg or a vegetarian savory. Stewed fruit or a baked apple may be taken for dessert.
- **Dinner:** A good-sized raw salad, of any suitable vegetable as obtainable, with whole wheat bread and butter, and prunes or other dried fruits as dessert.

Further short periods on the all-fruit diet should be undertaken at monthly intervals as required, for two or three consecutive days each time. The diet factor is of the supreme importance and fruits and salads must form the main basis of the future dietary. Alcohol, strong tea, coffee condiments, pickles and sauces should be avoided. Smoking, where habitual, should be given up.

Treatment through water is very beneficial in curing Hydrocele. Cold hip baths twice daily in the morning and the evening, for ten minutes each time, are especially valuable. For a cold hip bath, an ordinary tub may be used. It should be filled with cold water. The patient should sit in the tub, keeping the legs outside. A hot Epsom-salts bath is also very useful in the treatment of Hydrocele and should be taken once or twice weekly, where possible. Fresh air and outdoor exercise are vital to the success of this treatment. Sun and air bathing, where possible, should be undertaken. All habits and practices tending to lower the tone of the body should be studiously avoided; strain should be avoided as far as possible.

Chapter 40

Jaundice

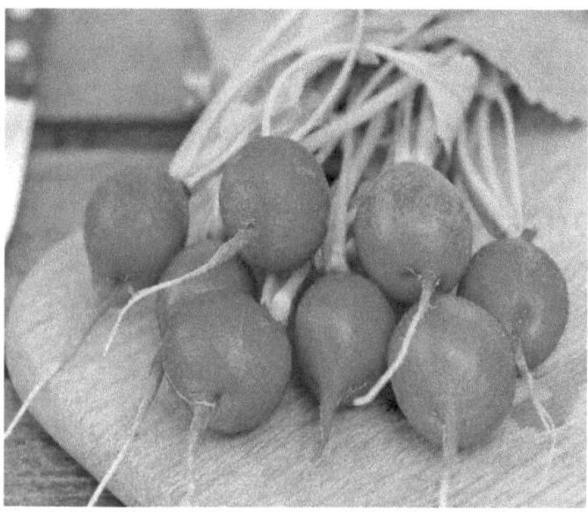

Natural remedy for jaundice in simple cases involves proper diet and exercise. However in serious cases, recovery is slow. The patient should take rest until the acute symptoms of the disease subside. The patient should be put on a fruit juice fast for a week. The juice of lemon, grapes, pear, carrot, beet, and sugarcane can be taken. A hot enema should be taken daily during the fast to ensure regular bowel elimination, thereby preventing the absorption of decomposed, poisonous material into the blood stream. Yoga asanas are also extremely helpful in the cure of jaundice.

The fruit juice fast may be discontinued after the severity of the disease is over and a simple diet may be resumed on the following lines:

- **Breakfast:** One fresh juicy fruit such as apple, papaya, grapes, berries and mangoes. One cup wheat dalia or one slice of whole wheat bread with a little butter.
- **Mid-morning:** Orange juice.
- **Lunch:** Two small chappatis of whole wheat flour, a cup of strained vegetable soup, a steamed leafy vegetable such as spinach, fenugreek or carrot and a glass of buttermilk.
- **Mid-afternoon:** Orange juice or coconut water.
- **Dinner:** Two whole wheat chappatis with a little ghee or butter, baked. Baked potato and one other leafy vegetable like spinach and fenugreek, a glass of hot milk with honey can be taken if desired.

Fats like ghee, butter, cream and oils must be avoided for at least two weeks, and after that their consumption should be kept down to the minimum. Digestive disturbances must be avoided. No food with an affinity to ferment or decompose in the lower intestines like pulses, legumes etc. should be included in diet. The juice of bitter luffa (karvi torai) is regarded as an effective (home) remedy for jaundice. The juice should be placed on the palm of the hand and drawn up through the nostrils. This will cause a profuse overflow of the yellow coloured fluid through the nostrils. The toxic matter having been evacuated in a considerable quantity, the patient will feel relieved.

Another valuable food therapy for jaundice is the green leaves of radish. The leaves should be pounded and their juices extracted through cloth. One pound of this juice daily is sufficient for an adult patient. It should be strained through a clean piece of muslin cloth before use. It provides instant relief. It induces a healthy appetite and proper evacuation of bowels, and this result in gradual decrease of the trouble. In most cases an absolute cure can be ensured within eight or ten days. Drinking a lot of water with lemon juice will guard the damaged liver cells. Alternate hot and cold compresses should be applied to the abdomen. A hot immersion bath at 104 degree Fahrenheit for ten minutes daily will be helpful in relieving the itching which sometimes accompanies jaundice and in the elimination of the bile pigment from the system through the skin and kidneys. Cold friction twice a day will be beneficial for general tone-up.

Certain asanas such as uthanpadasana, bhujangasana, viparita karani and shavasana, and anuloma-viloma, pranayama will be helpful in the treatment of jaundice. The jaundice patient can overcome the condition quite easily and build up his sick liver until it again functions normally with the above regime. With reasonable care in the diet and life style, and regular, restrained exercise and frequent exposure to sunshine and fresh air, a recurrence of liver trouble can be prevented.

Chapter 41

Neuritis

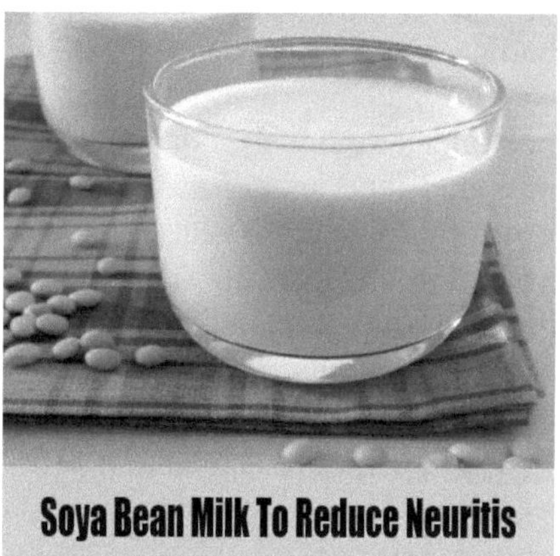

Soya Bean Milk To Reduce Neuritis

Natural cure of neuritis emphasises on the proper nutrition of the patient. The importance should be on whole grains, predominantly whole wheat, brown rice, raw and sprouted seeds, raw milk, particularly in soured form, and home made cottage cheese. In this regimen, the breakfast may consist of fresh fruits, a handful of raw nuts or a couple of tablespoons of sunflower and pumpkin seeds. Steamed vegetables, whole wheat, chappatis and a glass of butter-milk may be taken for lunch. The dinner may comprise a large bowl of fresh, green, vegetable salad, fresh home made cottage cheese, fresh butter and a glass of butter milk.

In severe cases, the patient should be put on a short juice fast for four or five days before being given the optimum diet. Carrot, beet, citrus fruits, apple and pineapple may be used for juices. All vitamins of the B group have proved extremely advantageous in the prevention and cure of neuritis. The disorder has been helped when vitamins B1, B2, B6, B12, and pantothenic acid have been given together, and tremendous pain, weakness and numbness in some cases have been relieved within an hour. The patient should avoid white bread, white sugar, refined cereals, meat, fish, tinned foods, tea, coffee, and condiments which are at the root of the trouble, by continuously flooding the tissues with acid impurities.

Certain remedies have been found very useful in the treatment of neuritis. One such therapy is soyabean milk. A cupful of soyabean milk mixed with a teaspoonful of honey should be taken every night in this condition. It tones up the nervous system due to its rich concentration of lecithin, vitamin B1 and glutanic acid. Soyabean milk is prepared by soaking the beans in water for about twelve hours. The skin of the beans is then removed and after a meticulous wash, they are turned into a fine paste in a grinding machine. The paste is mixed with water, three times its quantity. The milk should then be boiled on a slow fire, stirring it frequently. After it becomes little cooler, it should be strained through a cheese cloth and sugar added.

Barley brew is another useful remedy for neuritis. It is prepared by boiling one-quarter cup of all natural pearled barley in two quarters of water. When the water has boiled down to about one quarter, it should be strained cautiously. For better results, it should be mixed with butter-milk and lime juice. Raw carrot and spinach have proved helpful in neuritis as both these vegetables are rich in elements, the lack of which has led to this disease. The quickest and most effective way in which the body can attain and incorporate these elements is by drinking daily at least half a liter of the combined raw juices of carrot and spinach.

The patient should be given two or three hot Epsom-salt baths weekly. He should remain in the bath for twenty five to thirty minutes. The affected parts should also be bathed a number of times on a daily basis in the hot water containing Epsom salt. The patient should undertake walking and other moderate exercises.

Chapter 42

Psoriasis

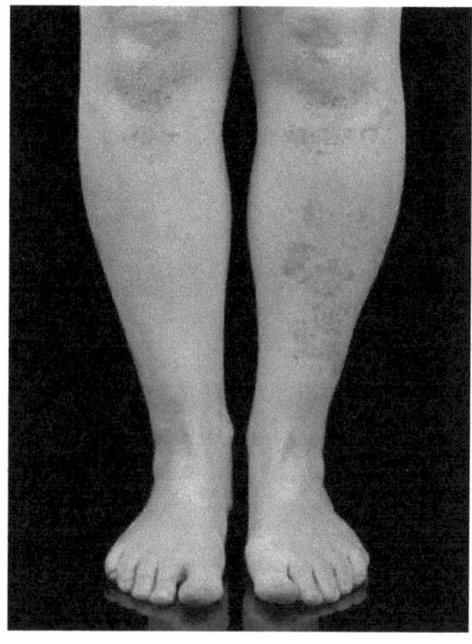

In the natural cure of psoriasis, a cleansing juice fast for about seven days is always desirable in the commencement of the treatment. Carrots, beats, cucumbers and grapes may be used for juices. Juices of citrus fruits should be avoided. The warm water enema should be used on a daily basis to cleanse the bowels during the fast. After the juice fast, the patient should take on the diet of three basic food groups, namely (i) seeds, nuts and grains, (ii) vegetables and (iii) fruits, with emphasis on raw seeds and nuts, particularly seasame seeds, pumpkin seeds, sunflower seeds and plenty of organically grown raw vegetables and fruits. All animal fats, including milk, butter and eggs should be avoided. Refined or processed foods and foods containing hydrogenated fats or white sugar, all condiments, tea and coffee, should also be avoided. After noticeable improvement, goat's milk, yogurt and home made cottage cheese may be added to the diet. Juice fasts may be repeated after four weeks on diet.

Vitamin E therapy has been found effective in the healing of psoriasis. Lecithin is considered a remarkable medication for psoriasis. In the form of granules, it may be taken four tablespoonfuls daily for two months. It may thereafter be reduced to two tablespoonfuls. Too frequent baths should be avoided. Soap should not be used. Regular sea water baths and application of sea water outwardly over the affected parts once a day are advantageous. The hot Epsom salts bath has proved valuable in psoriasis. Three full baths should be taken weekly until the trouble begins to subside. The number of baths thereafter may be reduced to two weekly and finally to one. The affected areas should also be bathed twice in hot water containing Epsom salt. After the bath a little olive oil may be applied. The skin should be kept completely clean by daily dry friction or sponge.

In many cases, psoriasis responds well to sunlight. The affected parts should be frequently exposed to the sun. The daily use of a sunlamp or ultra-violet light is also favourable. Cabbage leaves have been effectively used in the form of compresses in the treatment of psoriasis. The thickest and greenest outer leaves are most functional for use as compresses. They should be meticulously washed in warm water and dried with a towel. The leaves should be made flat, soft and smooth by rolling them with a rolling pin after removing the thick veins. They should be warmed and then applied efficiently to the affected part in an overlapping manner. A pad of soft wooden cloth should be put over it. The whole compress should then be secured with an elastic bandage.

The use of mud packs in the treatment of psoriasis is extremely beneficial. The packs are made by mixing the clay with a little water and applying to the affected areas. After the clay has dried, it is removed and fresh pack applied. Mud packs are eliminative in their action. They absorb and remove the toxins from the deceased areas. The patient should undertake plenty of regular exercise in fresh air, especially exposing the affected parts, and deep breathing exercises. He should keep away from all nervous tension and should have sufficient rest.

Chapter 43

Prostate Disorder

In the natural remedy of prostate disorder, the patient should abstain from all solid foods and live on water only for two or three days. The intake of water should be as plentiful as possible. Nothing should be added to the water except a little lemon juice, if desired. The water may be taken cold or hot and it should be taken every hour or so when awake. This will to a great extent augment the flow of urine. An enema may be taken once a day during fasting to clear the lower bowel of accumulations. After a systematic cleansing of the bowels, hot and cold applications may be used directly on the prostate gland and its surrounding parts. The heat relieves the tissues and a short cold immersion tones them up. The patient should take alternate hot and cold hip baths. These are of great value in relieving pain and reducing congestion.

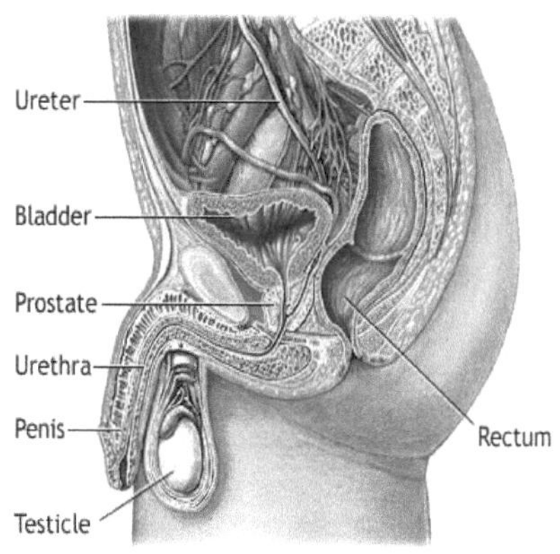

After the short fast, the patient should adopt an all-fruit diet for three days. The fruits should include apples, pears, oranges, grape-fruit, grapes, sweet limes, mangoes, melons and all other juicy fruits. This will help to clear toxins from the body and will also enable excess fat to be reduced to some extent. The exclusive fruit diet should be followed by a diet, consisting of two meals of fruits and one of cooked vegetables for further seven days. The vegetable meal should be taken in the evening and should consist of all kinds of cooked vegetables, preferably steam cooked. Thereafter, the patient may adopt a well-balanced diet of three basic food groups, namely (i) seeds, nuts and grains, (ii) vegetables and (iii) fruits.

The short lemon juice fast followed by an all-fruit diet and a further period on fruits and vegetables may be repeated after two or three months if required depending on the improvement being made. Pumpkin seeds have been found to be a successful home medication for prostate problems and many patients have been helped by their use. These seeds are rich in unsaturated fatty acids which are essential to the health of the prostate. Heavy starches, sweet stimulants and highly seasoned foods are totally forbidden, as they cause direct irritation on the prostate gland and bladder. The diet should also keep out spices, condiments, salt in excess, sauces, red meats, cheese, asparagus, watercress, greasy or fried foods, alcohol, tobacco and too much tea or coffee. The patient should avoid hurried meals and must chew his food thoroughly and slowly. Water should be taken between meals and not at mealtime.

The patient should avoid irregularities in eating and drinking, long periods of sitting and vigorous exercise. He should guard against constipation by taking plenty of fruits, bran and nuts. All efforts should be made to tone up the general condition of the body. With a general improvement in health, the condition will be greatly relieved.

Chapter 44

Hypoglycemia

In the natural remedy for hypoglycemia, seeds, nuts and grains should be the main constituents of the diet. Seeds and nuts should be taken in their raw form. Grains, in the form of cereals, should be cooked. Cooked grains are digested slowly and release sugar into the blood gradually six to eight hours after meals.

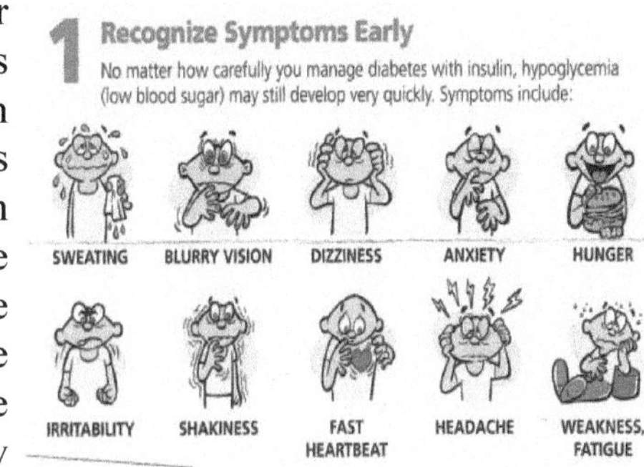

Persons suffering from low blood sugar should take six to eight small meals a day instead of two or three large ones. Eating raw nuts and seeds such as pumpkin or sunflower seeds or drinking milk, butter milk or fruit juices between meals will be extremely advantageous. All refined and processed foods, white sugar, white flour and their by products should be totally eliminated from the diet. Coffee, alcohol and soft drinks should also be avoided.

The following is the menu suggested for the patients of hypoglycemia.

- **Breakfast:** Nuts, seeds, fruit, cottage cheese and buttermilk.
- **Mid-morning:** Fruit, fruit juice or tomato juice.
- **Lunch:** Cooked cereals and milk.
- **Mid-afternoon:** A glass of fruit or vegetable juice or a snack consisting of nuts.
- **Dinner:** Vegetable salad with a cooked vegetable from among those allowed one or two slices of whole wheat bread, cottage cheese and butter milk.

Vegetables which can be taken in hypoglycemia are asparagus, beets, carrots, cucumbers, egg-plants, tomatoes, spinach, kale, lettuce, beans, and baked potatoes. Fruits which can be taken are apples, apricots, berries, peaches, and pineapples. Consumption of citrus fruits should be limited.

Foods rich in vitamin C, E and B-complex are very useful in the treatment of low blood sugar. Vitamins C and B increase tolerance to sugar and carbohydrates and help to normalise sugar metabolism. Pantothenic acid and vitamin B6 help to build up adrenals which are generally exhausted in persons with hypoglycemia. Vitamin E improves glycogen storage in the muscles and tissues. Proper rest is crucial for those suffering from low blood sugar. A peaceful mind is of extreme importance in this condition. Nervous strain and anxiety should be relieved by simple methods of meditation and relaxation. Yoga asanas like vakrasana, bhujangasana, halasana, sarbagasana and shavasana and pranayama like kapalbhati and anuloma-viloma will be beneficial.

Chapter 45

Sinusitis

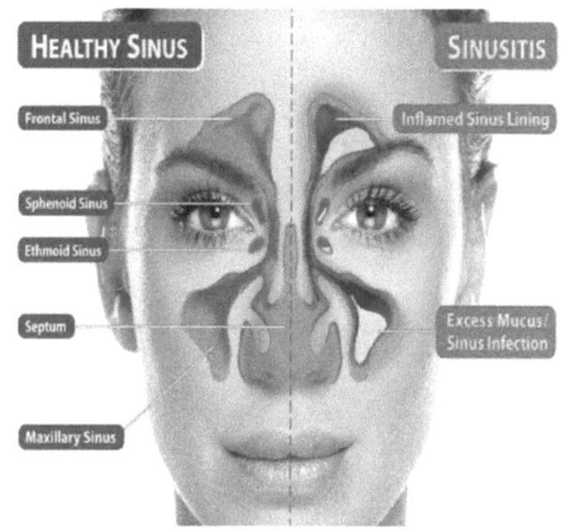

In natural remedy of sinusitis, the patient should take a balanced diet. Most persons with sinus trouble also suffer from acidity. Their diet should, therefore, turn to the alkaline side. The intake of salt should be reduced to the minimum as salt leads to accumulation of water in the tissues and expels calcium from the body. In the acute stage of the disease, when fever is present, the patient should abstain from all solid foods and only drink fresh fruit and vegetable juices diluted with water. After fever subsides, he may adopt a low-calorie raw fruit and vegetable diet with plenty of raw juices.

After the acute symptoms are over, the patient may gradually embark upon a well-balanced diet of three basic food groups, namely seeds, nuts and grains; vegetables and fruits. In persistent chronic conditions, repeated short juice fasts may be undertaken for a week or so at intervals of two months. Those suffering from sinusitis should completely avoid fried and starchy foods, white sugar, white flour, rice, macaroni products, pies, cakes and candies. They should also avoid strong spices, meat and products. Butter and ghee should be used sparingly. Honey should be used for sweetening. All cooked foods should be freshly prepared for each meal. Vegetables should be taken in liberal quantities. All kinds of fruits can be taken with the exception of those belonging to citrus group such as lemon, lime, orange and grapefruit. Milk should be taken in liberal quantities as it contains calcium which has a marked effect in overcoming inflammation of the tissues.

A diet rich in vitamin A is the best insurance against cold and sinus trouble. Some of the valuable sources of this vitamin are whole milk, curds, egg yolk, pumpkin, carrot, leafy vegetables, tomato, oranges, mango and papaya. One of the most effective remedies for sinus problems is to eat pungent herbs like garlic and onion which tend to break up mucous congestion all through the respiratory tract. One should begin with small mild doses and increase them gradually. Beneficial results can also be achieved by adding these herbs in moderate amounts to regular meals. Carrot juice used separately or in combination with juices of beet and cucumber or with spinach juice is highly beneficial in the treatment of sinus trouble. 100 ml. each of beet and cucumber juice or 200 ml. of spinach juice should be mixed with 300 ml. of carrot juice in these combinations.

Cold application over the sinus will give great relief; alternate hot and cold applications will also prove beneficial. Yoga asanas such as viparit karani, bhujangasana, yogamudra and shavasana, yogic kriyas, such as jalneti and sutraneti and pranayamas like anuloma-viloma and suryabhedan will be beneficial in the treatment of sinus trouble. Plenty of sleep, adequate rest and fresh air are essential in the treatment of sinus trouble. Patients should avoid the use of perfumes and strongly scented hair oil.

Chapter 46

Weight Gain

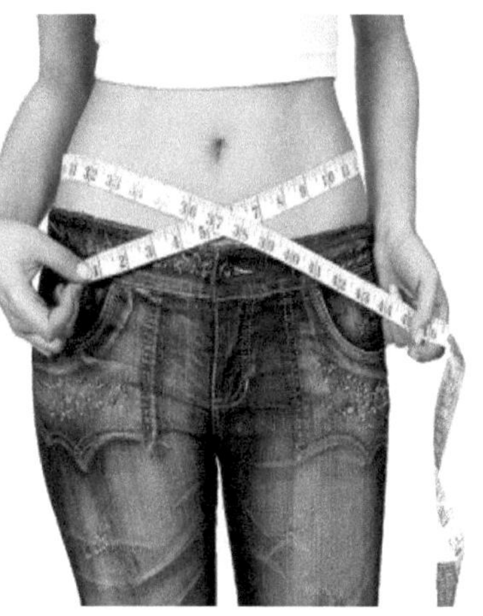

Diet plays an important role in building up health for gaining weight in the natural remedy for weight loss. Nutrients which help keep the nerves relaxed are of extreme importance as nervousness causes all the muscles to become stressed and the energy which goes into the tenseness inefficiently uses up a great deal of food. Although all vitamins and minerals are required for a sound health, the most important ones are vitamin D and B6, calcium and magnesium. The richest sources of vitamin D are milk, cod liver oil and the rays of the sun. Calcium is also supplied by milk and yogurt. Magnesium can be obtained from green leafy vegetables such as spinach, radish, parsley, turnip, and beet tops.

Lack of appetite can result from an insufficient supply of vitamin B, which leads to low production of hydrochloric acid by the stomach. Hydrochloric acid is vital for the digestion of food and absorption of vitamins and minerals into the blood. It is, therefore, necessary that the daily diet should be rich in vitamin B for normal appetite. Foods rich in vitamin B are all whole grain cereals, soyabean, eggs, blackstrap molasses, nuts and butter. Vegetable oil is of unique value to those wishing to gain weight as it is rich in vitamin E and necessary fatty acids.

Underweight persons should eat frequent small meals as they tend to feel full quickly. Meals may be divided into six small ones instead of three big ones. These may consist of three smaller meals and three substantial snacks between them. The weight building quality of a food is measured by the number of calories it contains. To gain weight, the diet should comprise of more calories than are used in daily activities so as to allow the surplus to be stored as body fat. Excessive intake of refined carbohydrates and fats may help the individual to put on weight but this will be disadvantageous to general health. Beverages containing caffeine like soft drinks, coffee and tea should be curtailed. Smoking should be given up. Water should not be taken with meals but half an hour before or one hour after meals.

An exclusive milk diet for rapid gain of weight has been advocated by some nature cure practitioners. In the commencement of this mode of treatment, the patient should fast for three days on warm water and like juice so as to cleanse the system. Subsequently, he should have a glass of milk every two hours from 8 a.m. to 8 p.m. the first day, a glass every hour and half the next day, and a glass every hour the third day. Then the quantity of milk should be steadily increased so as to take a glass every half an hour from 8 a.m. to 8 p.m. The milk should be fresh and should be sipped very slowly through a straw. Figs are an exceptional food remedy for increasing weight in case of thinness.

Regular exercises like walking and dancing, yoga, meditation and massage are also imperative as they serve as relaxants, lessen anxiety and stimulate good sleep. Yoga asanas which will be especially helpful are sarvangasana, halasana and matsyasana. A balanced diet together with adequate exercise, rest, emotional balance and the absence of acute diseases will facilitate an underweight person to build a healthy body and to put on weight.

Chapter 47

Menstrual Disorders

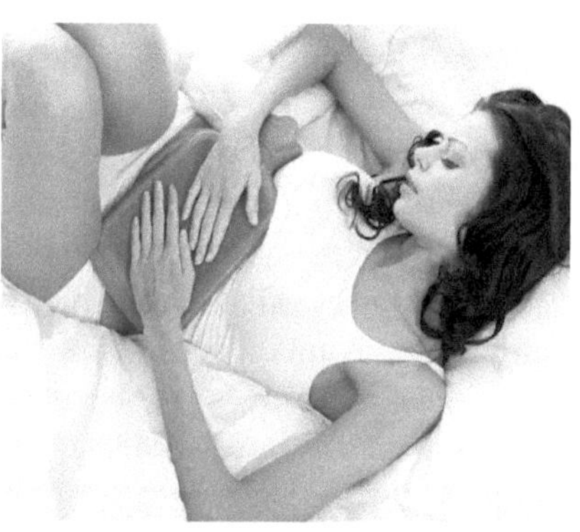

In the natural therapy for Menstrual Disorders, the sufferer should begin with an all fruit diet for about five days. In this course of therapy, the patient should have three meals a day of fresh, juicy fruits, such as apples, pears, pineapple, grapes, papaya, oranges, peaches and melon. No other food should be taken; otherwise the significance of the entire treatment will be lost. During this period the bowels should be cleansed on a daily basis with a warm water enema.

After the all-fruit diet, the sufferer should adopt a well balanced diet on the following lines:

- **Upon rising:** A glass of lukewarm water should be mixed with the freshly squeezed juice of half a lime and a spoon of honey.
- **Breakfast:** Fresh fruits such as apple, papaya, banana, orange, grapes and milk.
- **Lunch:** A bowl of freshly prepared steamed vegetable such as carrot, cauliflower, and beans, cabbage, two or three whole wheat chappatis.
- **Dinner:** A large bowl of fresh green vegetable salad with all obtainable vegetable such as carrot, tomatoes, radish, cabbage, cucumber, red beets and onion and sprouts.

The diet factor is of the extreme importance. Fruits and salads, nature's body-cleansing and health-restoring foods, must constitute the bulk of the future diet along with whole grains, nuts and seeds, particularly in sprouted forms. Frequent small meals should be taken instead of few large ones to avoid low blood sugar which is common at the time of menstruation. The foods which should be avoided in future are white-flour products, sugar, and confectionery, rich cakes, flesh foods, pastries, sweets, refined cereals, rich, heavy, or greasy foods, tinned or preserved foods, strong tea, coffee, pickles, condiments and sauces. Smoking, if habitual, should be given up entirely as it aggravates menstrual disorders.

A further short period on all -fruit, say two or three consecutive days can be undertaken at monthly intervals, according to the need of the case. The morning dry friction and cold hip baths should form a habitual feature of the cure. All cold baths should however, be suspended at the time of the menstrual period. Certain remedies have been found useful in menstrual disorders. Cooked banana flower eaten with curd is one of the more important of such remedies. The banana flower appears to amplify progesterone hormone and lessen the bleeding. Beet juice has been found very effectual for menstrual disorders. Coriander seeds are extremely advantageous in the treatment of excessive menstruation. Ginger has been useful in menstrual disorders. Sesame seeds are also useful in menstrual disorders. Its regular use, two days prior to the expected periods, cures insufficient menstruation. Warm hip bath containing a handful of bruised sesame seeds should be at the same time taken along with this receipt. Safflower seeds have also been found to be valuable in the treatment of painful menstruation.

Chapter 48

Leucorrhoea

In the natural remedy for Leucorrhoea, first and foremost the body should be free from all the accumulated toxins. Proper diet, adequate sleep, exercise, fresh air and sunshine are indispensable part of the treatment. To start with, the patient should fast for three or four days on lemon water or fruit juices for the removal of the morbid matter from the body. During this period the bowel should be cleansed on a daily basis with a lukewarm water enema. In case of habitual constipation, steps should be taken for its eradication. Subsequent to a short fast, the patient may take up an all fruit-diet for about a week. In this course of therapy, she should have three meals a day of fresh juicy fruits such as grapefruit, oranges, pineapple, apples, pears, grapes, and peaches. If the patient is suffering from anemia, or is too thin, the diet may consist of fruits and milk. The patient may then slowly but surely embark upon a well-balanced diet consisting of three basic food groups specifically (i) seeds, nuts and grains, (ii) fruits and (iii) vegetables.

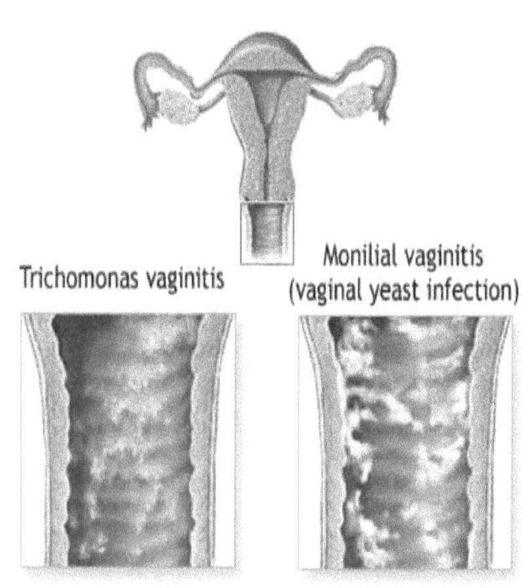

Fresh fruits or fruit juices only should be taken between meals. All forms of white four, white sugar, fried and greasy foods, preserves, tea and coffee should be avoided. An effective home tonic for leucorrhoea is lady's finger. Fenugreek seeds are another exceptional home remedy for leucorrhoea. They should be taken internally in the form of tea and also used as a douche. Water therapy is enormously advantageous in curing leucorrhoea. A cold hip bath twice a day for ten minutes will help relieve congestion in the pelvic region and smooth the progress of quick elimination of morbid matter.

In severe cases of leucorrhoea, the douche should be done daily. The passive inflammation of the affected organs can be cured by regular hot hip baths at 40 o C for ten minutes and normal use of wet girdle pack for ninety minutes every night. Yoga asanas, in particular those which improve muscles of the abdomen and uterus are extremely beneficial and should be practiced on a regular basis. These asanas are paschimottanasana, padmasana, bhujansana, sarvagasana, halasana and salabhasana. The patient should fully relax and should avoid mental anxiety and worry. Abdominal exercises and walking are also helpful.

Chapter 49

Prolapse of Uterus

Natural Remedy for the Prolapse of the uterus should aim at building up the internal musculature of the body. Proper diet and exercises are of supreme importance in the natural cure of displaced womb. Any propensity towards tight lacing, constant stooping, and heavy lifting must be cautiously guarded against, once a normal regime is undertaken, as these will involuntarily tend to hold up the success of the treatment. The patient should adopt an all-fruit diet for about five days at the beginning of the treatment. During this period she should take three meals consisting of juicy fruits such as apple, orange, pineapple, grapes at five hourly intervals. The bowel should be cleansed on a daily basis with a warm water enema. After the all fruit diet , the patient should steadily embark upon a well-balanced diet, based on three basic food groups, namely, (i) seeds, nuts and grains (ii) vegetables and (iii) fruits.

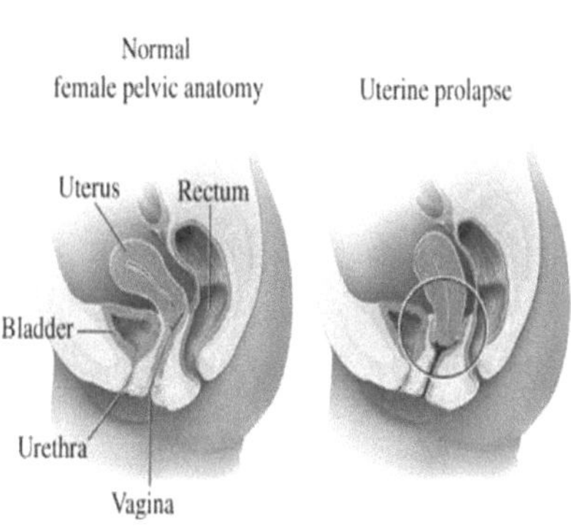

The all fruit diet should be repeated for three days at monthly intervals till the condition improves. Carrots have proved functional in the treatment of Prolapse of the uterus. For Prolapse of the uterus, pulped carrots should be placed in a muslin bag and inserted in a vagina. This should be kept for some time using fresh carrots every twelve hours. This will heal and strengthen the parts and help to a great extent in preventing any further disorders in the female reproductive system. A hot Epsom salts bath is also valuable in the treatment of Prolapse of the uterus and should be undertaken twice a week. No soaps should be used with the bath as it will hinder the favourable effects. The alternate hot and cold hip baths are also helpful and should be undertaken at night on alternate days.

Exercises to toughen the pelvic musculature are exceptionally useful in the treatment of Prolapse of the uterus. Lying on a couch with the legs elevated than the rest of the body is very helpful in relieving pain and uneasiness from a displaced womb. This should be done from half an hour to an hour two or three times on a daily basis. The patient should also carry out other exercises aimed at strengthening the abdominal muscles. These exercises will help to a large extent in correcting the displacement of the uterus. Women should always take precautions to space out their children so as to prevent repeated successive deliveries. This will allow the genital issues to regain their strength and energy and thereby thwart Prolapse of the uterus.

Chapter 50

Goitre

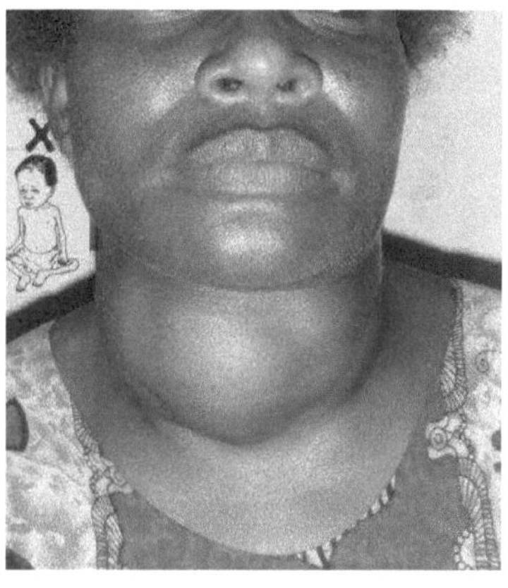

Natural remedy for goitre prescribes the cleansing of the system, a proper food habit, rest and relaxation. To begin with, juices of fruits such as orange, apple, pineapple and grapes may be taken every two or three hours from 8 a.m. to 8 p.m. for five days. The bowels should be cleansed on a daily basis with lukewarm water. After the juice fast, the patient may spend a further three days on fruits and milk, taking three meals a day of juicy fruits, such as apple, papaya, pineapple, grapes with a glass of milk, at five hourly intervals. Subsequently, a balanced diet on the following line may be adopted:

- **Breakfast:** Fresh acid foods such as apples, grapes, grapefruit, oranges, pears, a glass of whole milk and a handful of raw nuts.
- **Mid-morning:** A glass of fruit or vegetable juice to which a table- spoon of yeast has been added.
- **Lunch:** Steamed vegetables, whole wheat chappatis and a glass of buttermilk.
- **Mid-afternoon:** A glass of milk or fruit juice.
- **Dinner:** Vegetable soup, a large bowl of salad of raw vegetables in season such as lettuce, tomato, and celery, sprouts such as alfalfa seeds and mung beans and home made cottage cheese or nuts.

The patient should take ample rest and spend a day in bed every week for the first two months of the treatment. More and more exercise should be taken after the symptoms settle. The appetite of the thyroid patient is generally very large and the weight reduction cannot be prevented for some time. This is because until the heart beat slows down and the tremors stop, there will be incomplete assimilation of the food. But as soon as the balance is restored, weight will slowly amplify. As weight increases, the almost constant hunger will slowly but surely disappear; on no account should any stimulants be administered to create an appetite.

Certain foods and fluids are exceptionally injurious to the goitre patients and this should be avoided by them. These consist of white flour products, white sugar, flesh foods, preserves, condiments, fried or greasy foods, tea, coffee and alcohol. No drugs should be taken as they cause irritation in the tissues. Iodine is unquestionably most helpful in many cases. But it should be introduced in organic form. All foods containing iodine should be taken generously. These are asparagus, pineapple, whole rice, cabbage, carrots, garlic, onion, oats, tomatoes, watercress, and strawberries. Great care must be taken never to allow the body to become exhausted and any irritation likely to cause emotional distress should be avoided.

Strict obedience to a suitable diet is indispensable for complete cure. Daily intake of food should consist of fresh fruits and vegetables and the starch elements should be confined to whole wheat products and potatoes. Potatoes are the most valuable form of starch. They should if possible be taken in their jackets. The protein foods should be confined to peas, beans, lentils, eggs, cheese and nuts. Milk and all flesh proteins must be avoided. The diet outlines here should be firmly adhered to for a year, and the compresses on the neck and the waist applied for five consecutive nights in a week for two months and discontinued for one month.

Water treatments should be taken to increase skin elimination. Application of a sponge to the entire body before retiring and a cold sponge on rising will be very helpful. It is most important that the bowels are kept working proficiently to avoid danger of a toxic condition of the blood arising from that source. All efforts should be made to prevent emotional anxiety. There may be a light recurrence of this enormously nervous complaint for some time, but the attacks will become less severe and of shorter duration as the treatment progresses.

Chapter 51

Hiatus Hernia

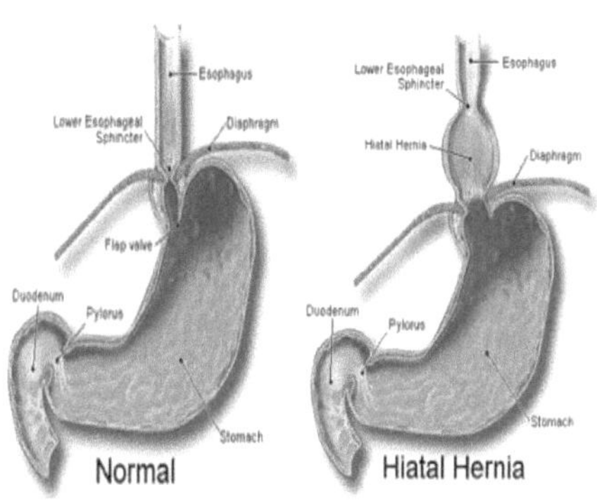

In the natural remedy for hiatus hernia it is advisable to raise the head end of the bed by placing bricks below the legs of the bed. This will prevent the regurgitation of food during the night. The next vital step towards treating hiatus hernia is relaxation. An important measure in this direction is diaphragmatic breathing. It is important to be able to relax at any time and in that way prevent building up of physical and mental tensions which may cause actual physical symptoms. The best method for this is practice shavasana.

The patient of hiatus hernia should observe certain precautions in their eating habits. The most important amongst these is not to take water with meals, but half an hour before or one hour after a meal. This helps the digestive process significantly and reduces the frequency of heart burn. Drinking water with meals increases the overall weight in the stomach, slows down the digestive process by diluting the digestive process and this increases the risk of fermentation and gas formation, which distends the stomach and causes uneasiness and pain.

Another important factor in the treatment of this disease is to take frequent small meals instead of three large ones. Thorough mastication of foods is also important, both to break up the food into small particles and to slow down the rate of intake. The diet of the patient should consist of seeds, vegetables and fruits, nuts and whole cereal grains, with emphasis on fresh fruits, raw or lightly cooked vegetables and sprouted seeds. The foods which should be avoided are over processed foods like white bread and sugar, cakes and biscuits, rice puddings and over cooked vegetables. At least 50 per cent of the diet should include fruits and vegetables, and the remaining fifty per cent of protein, carbohydrates and fat.

Raw juices extracted from fresh fruits and vegetables are helpful in hiatus hernia, and the patient should take these juices half an hour before each meal. Carrot juice is in particular advantageous as it has a very restorative effect, and is rich in vitamin A and calcium. It is an alkaline food which soothes the stomach. All juices should be diluted with water. The hot drinks should always be allowed to cool a little before taking. Extremes in temperature, in both food and drink should be avoided; drinks should not be taken hurriedly, but sipped little by little. The patient should keep away from condiments, pickles, strong tea, coffee, alcoholic beverages and smoking.

Chapter 52

Whooping Cough

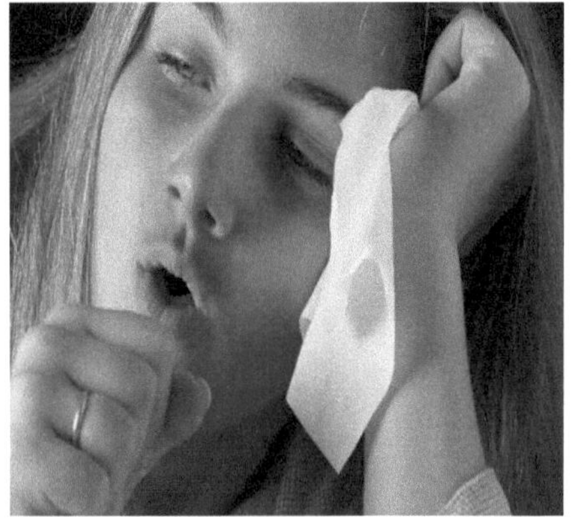

Natural remedy for whooping cough begins with the patient being placed on a fast, on orange juice and water for few days. He should be given the juice of an orange diluted with warm water. He should not be given milk or anything else. He should be given tepid water enema on a daily basis during this period to cleanse the bowels. In case of constipation, a mild laxative, if possible castor oil should be administered. This will also reduce the pain in the abdominal muscles which are generally strained during the paroxysms of coughing. Cold packs should be applied to the throat and upper chest as required. Epsom salt baths will be favourable during this period. After the more sever symptoms have cleared, the patient should be placed on an exclusive diet of fresh fruits for a few days. In this course of therapy, one should take fresh juicy fruits such as pineapple, apple, orange and papaya. After further recuperation, he can take on a regular well balanced diet, according to his age. The emphasis should be on fresh fruit, fruit and vegetable juices and milk.

When the restorative stage has been reached, the patient should be encouraged to spend as much time as possible out of doors. Certain home remedies have been found advantageous in the treatment of whooping cough. The most successful of these remedies is the use of garlic. The syrup of garlic should be given in the dosage of five drops to a tablespoon two or three times a day for treating this condition. It should be given more often if the coughing spells are recurrent and violent. Ginger is another helpful medication for whooping cough. A teaspoon of fresh ginger juice, mixed with a cup of fenugreek (methi) decoction and honey to taste, is an excellent diaphoretic. It acts as an expectorant in this disease. Syrup prepared by mixing a teaspoon of fresh radish (muli) with equal quantity of honey and a little rock salt, is valuable in the healing of this disease. It should be given thrice on a daily basis. Almond (badam) oil is valuable in whooping cough. It should be given mixed with ten drops each of fresh white onion juice and ginger juice, on a daily basis thrice for a fortnight. It will provide relief to the patient.

Chapter 53

Mumps

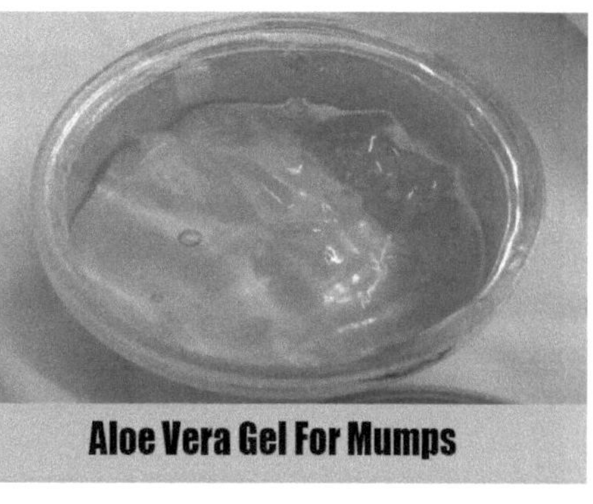

Aloe Vera Gel For Mumps

Natural remedy for mumps calls for the patient to be put in bed for several days until the temperature returns to normal. He should be kept on a diet of orange juice diluted with tepid water for a few days. If the orange juice does not suit, the juices of other fruits such as apple, pineapple, grapes, or vegetables like carrot should be given. The lukewarm water enema should be used on a daily basis during this period. Hot and cold fomentations should be applied every two hours during the day for about ten minutes, and should consist of two or three hot applications, followed by a cold one. The mouth should be cleaned with an antiseptic wash. When the patient can swallow food at ease and the swelling has subsided, an all fruit diet should be adopted for a day or two. Subsequently, he may be allowed to gradually embark upon a well balanced diet of natural foods, with emphasis on fresh fruits and raw vegetables.

Chebulic myroblen (harad or haritaki) is one of the most successful remedies for mumps. A thick paste should be made from this herb by rubbing in water and applied over the swelling. It will give relief. The leaves of the peepul tree are one more valuable home remedy for this disease. The leaves should be smeared with ghee and warmed over a fire. They should then be bandaged over the inflammed part, with advantageous results. The use of the herb Indian aloe (ghee kunwar or musabhar) is a well known medication for inflammed and painful part of the body in the indigenous system of medicine. A piece of a leaf of this herb should be peeled on one side and sprinkled with a little turmeric (haldi) and extract of Indian barberry (rasaut) and bandaged over the swelling after warming.

The seeds of asparagus (halon) are valuable in mumps. These seeds combined with the seeds of fenugreek (methi) should be ground together to a consistency of a paste. This paste can be applied beneficially over the swelling. The dry ginger (adrak) is considered beneficial in the treatment of mumps. It should be made into a paste and applied over the swollen parts. As the paste dries, the swelling will be reduced and the pain will also settle. The leaves of margosa or neem are also functional in the treatment of mumps. The leaves of this tree and turmeric (haldi) should be made into a paste and applied externally over the affected parts. It will bring good results.

Chapter 54

Cystitis

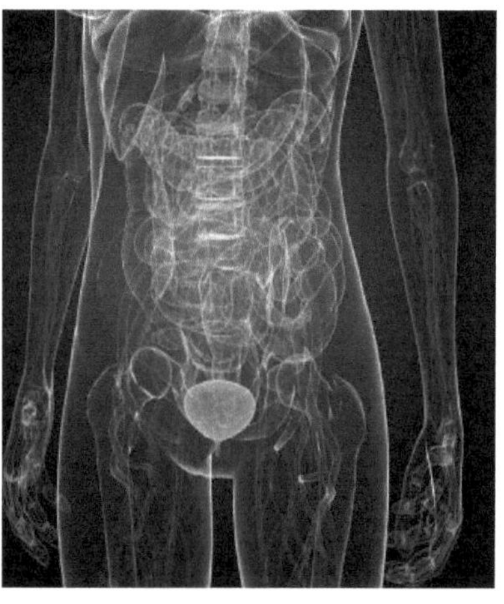

Natural remedy of acute cystitis involves withholding all solid food without delay. If there is fever, the patient should fast either on water or tender coconut water for three or four days. If there is no fever, raw vegetable juices, particularly carrot juice diluted with water, should be taken every two or three hours. By so doing the biochemical energy needed for digestion and metabolism of food is diverted to the process of eliminating toxins and promoting curing and repair. It is wise to rest and keep warm at this time. Pain can be relieved by immersing the pelvis in hot water or alternatively by applying heat to the abdomen, using a towel wrung out in hot water, covering it with dry towel to maintain warmth. Care should be taken to keep away from scalding. A little vegetable oil smoothly rubbed into the skin, will avoid too much reddening. This treatment may be continued for three or four days, by which time the inflammation should have subsided and the temperature returned to normal.

For the next two or three days, only ripe sub acid fruits may be taken three or four times on a daily basis. These fruits may include peaches, apples, grapes, pears, and melon, as available. While the hot compresses are intended to mitigate pain, the use of cold water compresses to the abdomen is most helpful, if correctly applied, in relieving pelvic congestion and increasing the activity of the skin. Care should, however, be taken to make sure that compresses do not cause chilling. After the all fruit diet, the patient may steadily embark upon a well balanced diet, consisting of seeds, nuts and grains, vegetables and fruits. The patient should keep away from refined carbohydrates and salt, both at table and in cooking. Salt disturbs the balance of electrolytes and tends to raise blood pressure, which is commonly already raised in kidney troubles.

The prescribed dietary should keep out meat, fish and poultry. They produce uric acid. Most cases of food poisoning and infections, which may lead to gastritis and colitis, are also caused by the flesh foods. In case of chronic cystitis, the patient should begin the treatment of strict observance to the dietary programme, designed to cleanse the blood and other tissues and at the same time provide a rich source of natural vitamins and minerals in balanced proportions. The patient may take on the following restricted diet for seven to ten days.

- **Upon arising:** A glass of unsweetened apple juice or carrot juice
- **Breakfast:** Fresh fruits, selected mainly from apple, pear, peach grapes, melon, and pineapple and a glass of buttermilk, sweetened with a little honey.
- **Mid-morning:** Tender coconut water.
- **Lunch:** A salad of raw vegetables such as carrot, beetroot and cabbage, mixed with curd and a tablespoon of honey.
- **Mid-afternoon:** One cup of unsweetened grape juice.
- **Dinner:** A salad of green leafy vegetables and a fresh fruit, preferably a portion of melon sweetened with a teaspoon of honey.

Subsequent to the restricted diet, the patient should slowly embark on a well balanced diet, consisting of seed, nuts and grains, vegetables and fruits. Even after the recuperation from the chronic condition, it will be prudent for the individual to live exclusively on vegetables or on tender coconut water or raw vegetable juices for a day or two, every month. The water therapy and other health building methods should, however, are continued to the greatest extent possible, so that the patient may stay cured.

Chapter 55

Pneumonia

In the beginning of the natural remedy for Pneumonia, the patient should be kept on a diet of raw juices for five to ten days, depending on the severity of the disease. In this course of therapy he should take a glass of fruit or vegetable juice diluted with warm water every two or three hours. Fruits such as apple, pineapple, orange, mosambi and grapes and vegetables like carrots, tomatoes may be used for juices. After a diet of raw juices, when the fever subsides, the patient should three or four more days on an exclusive fresh fruit diet, taking three meals a day of juicy fruits such as pineapple, mangoes, apple, grapes, orange, lemon and papaya. Subsequently, he may steadily take up a well balanced diet of natural foods consisting of foods, seeds, and grains, vegetables and fruits with emphasis on fresh fruits and raw vegetables.

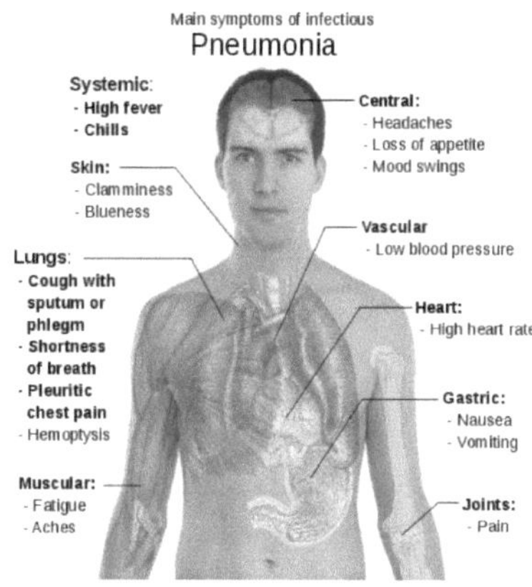

The patients should be given warm enema on a daily basis to cleanse the bowel during the period of raw juice therapy and all fruit diet and thereafter, when required. The patient should avoid strong tea, coffee, refined foods, fried foods, white sugar, white flour and all products made from them, condiments and pickles. He should also keep away from all meats as well as alcoholic beverages and smoking. Sipping of cold water has also been found useful in the treatment of pneumonia. The patient should sip cold water at short intervals so long as the fever continues. The cold water is cooling to the feverish blood. Certain home remedies have been found beneficial in the treatment of pneumonia. During the early acute stage of this disease, herbal tea made from fenugreek seeds will help the body to produce perspiration, drive out toxicity and cut down the period of fever.

During this treatment, no other food or nourishment should be taken as fasting and fenugreek will allow the body to correct these respiratory problems in a few days. Garlic juice can also be applied externally to the chest with useful results as it is an irritant. Sesame seeds (til) are valuable in pneumonia. An infusion of the seeds, mixed with a tablespoon of linseed, a pinch of common salt and a desert spoon of honey, should be given in the cure of this disease. This will help eliminate catarrhal matter and phlegm from the bronchial-tubes. The pain of pneumonia can be relieved by rubbing oil of turpentine over the rib cage and wrapping warmed cotton wool over it.

Chapter 56

Premature Greying of Hair

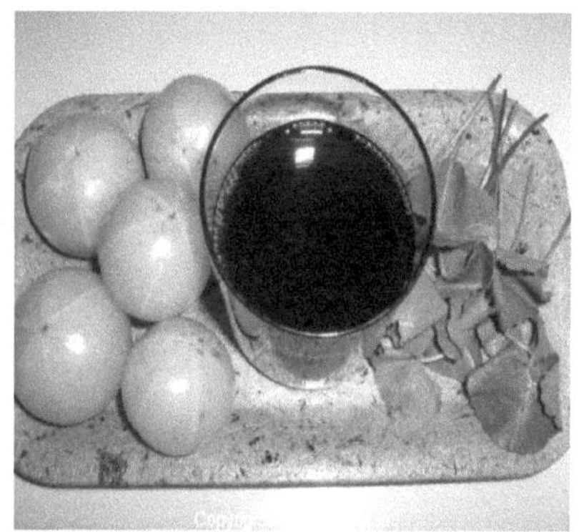

In naturopathy, diet is of supreme significance in the natural remedy to prevent and cure the premature greying of hair. The vitamins considered functional to prevent premature greying of hair are pantothenic acid, para- aminobenzoic acid and inositol. To gain satisfactory results, all three of these vitamins, belonging to B group, should be supplied at one time if possible in a form which gives all B vitamins, such as yeast, wheat germ and liver. Drinking a litre of yogurt on a daily basis with a tablespoon of yeast before each meal will be an admirable medication for the prevention and treatment of premature greying of hair.

Carrots are in particular useful in furnishing fresh blood and maintaining the health of the hair. Certain home remedies have been found valuable in the prevention and treatment of premature greying of hair. The foremost among these is the use of Indian gooseberry or amla which is an important hair tonic for enriching hair growth and hair pigmentation. The fruit, cut into pieces, should be dried, preferably in the shade. These pieces should be boiled in coconut oil till the solid matter become little charred dust. This darkish oil is very useful in preventing greying. The water in which dried amla pieces are soaked overnight is considered exceedingly advantageous in the treatment of premature greying of hair. This water should be used for the last rinse while washing the hair.

Massaging the scalp with a teaspoonful of amla juice mixed with a teaspoonful of almond oil or few drops of lime juice, every night has proved useful in the prevention and treatment of premature greying of hair. Liberal intake of curry leaves is considered beneficial in preventing premature greying of hair. These have the property to give vivacity and strength to hair roots. New hair roots that grow are healthier with normal pigment. The leaves can be used in the form of chutney or these may be squeezed in buttermilk or lassi. When the leaves are boiled in coconut oil, the oil forms an outstanding hair tonic to encourage hair growth and bring back hair pigmentation. The butter made from cow's milk has the property to prevent premature greying of hair.

Jhingaka or Ribbed gourd, known as torai in the vernacular, boiled in coconut oil is another effective medication for premature greying of hair. Pieces of this vegetable should be dried in the shade. These dried pieces should be soaked in coconut oil and kept aside for three or four days. The oil should then be boiled till the solid is reduced to a blackened deposit. The paste of henna leaves, boiled in coconut oil to get darkish oil, can be used as a hair dye to blacken grey hair. The paste itself can be applied to the hair and washed away after a few hours to dye the grey hair. Washing the hair with concentrated tea extract twice a week is also considered functional in colouring grey hair to brown or black.

Chapter 57

Female Sterility

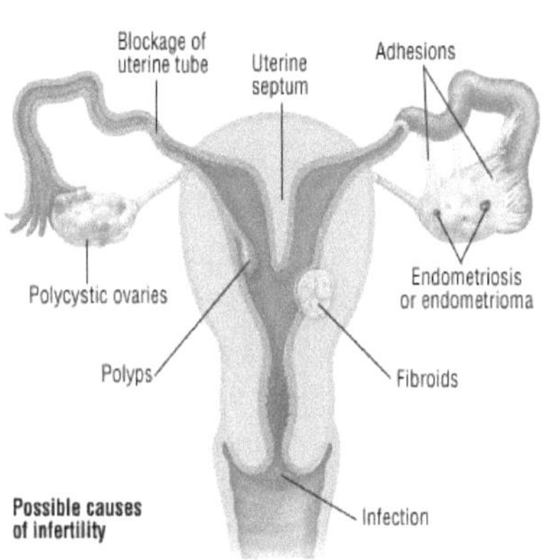

Possible causes of infertility

Natural remedy for female sterility is to undertake a fasting therapy which is the best remedy for the treatment of disorders resulting from toxins in the system. A short fast of two or three days should be undertaken at normal intervals by women who are not capable to bear children. The bowels should be cleansed by a lukewarm water enema during the period of fasting and afterwards when required. This will have an advantageous effect not only on the digestive system but also on the surrounding organs of the urinary and genital system. Diet is the most vital aspect in the treatment of sterility. It should consist of three basic health building food groups namely (i) seeds, nuts and grains, (ii) vegetables and (iii) fruits. These foods should be supplemented with milk, vegetable oils and honey. The best way to take milk is in its soured form that is curd and cottage cheese. Each food group should more or less form the bulk of one of three meals.

Sprouting is an exceptional way of consuming seeds, beans and grains in their raw form. In the process of sprouting, the nutritional value is multiplied, new vitamins are created and the protein quality is improved.

The daily menu of a health building and vitalising diet may be on the following lines:

- **Upon rising:** A glass of lukewarm water with a juice of half a lemon and a spoonful of honey.
- **Breakfast:** Fresh fruits like orange, banana, apple, grapes and grapefruit and a glass of milk.

- **Lunch:** A bowl of steamed vegetables seasoned with vegetable oil or butter and salt, two or three whole wheat chappatis and a glass of buttermilk.
- **Mid-afternoon:** A glass of fresh fruit or vegetable juice. Dinner: A large bowl of salad made up of fresh vegetables such as carrots, beetroots and onion, tomatoes, and sprouted moong or bengal gram.
- **Bed-time:** A glass of milk or an apple.

Too much of fat, spicy foods, strong white sugar, white flour, refined cereals, tea, coffee, flesh foods, greasy or fried foods should all be avoided. Certain nutrients, in particular vitamin C and E and zinc have been found helpful in some cases of sterility. Certain remedies have also been found functional in the treatment of female sterility where there are no organic defects or congenital deformities. One such therapy is a tender root of the banyan tree. These roots should be dried in the shade and finally powdered. This powder should be mixed five times their weight with milk and taken at night for three consecutive nights after the monthly periods are over. No other food should be taken with this. It should be repeated after the completion of menstrual cycle every month till conception takes place.

An infusion of the fresh tender leaves of jambul fruit (jamun) taken with honey or buttermilk, is an excellent medication for sterility and miscarriage due to ovarian or endometrium functional disorders. The leaves most probably encourage the secretion of progesterone hormone and help the absorption of vitamin E. The eggplant is also helpful in overcoming functional sterility. Cooked tender eggplants should be eaten with butter-milk everyday for a month or two for this purpose. It increases the capacity to take up vitamin E and stimulate the secretion of progesterone. Other helpful measures in overcoming female sterility are mud packs and cold water treatment like a hip bath and a wet girdle pack. These treatments will significantly improve internal circulation in the genital organs and will relieve them of all kinds of inflammation and other abnormalities. Mud packs may be applied to the abdomen and sexual organs.

Certain yoga asanas which assist tone up the gonads should be practiced on a regular basis for overcoming female sterility. These asanas are sarvagasana, matyasana, ardha matsyendrasana, paschimottanasana, and salabhasana. All these practices together with clean habits, proper rest and relaxation will go a long way in overcoming female sterility.

Chapter 58

Allergies

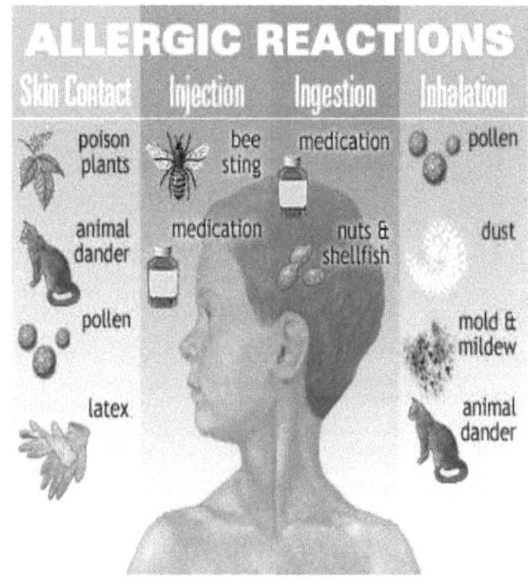

In naturopathy, there are a number of natural remedies for allergies. Firstly, the sources must be identified. This is a complicated method but not an impossible task. Secondly, once the sources are discovered, they should be kept away from. Thirdly, and most importantly, general health and resistance should be built up to establish immunity to them. There are two methods to become aware of disturbing foods. The first method is the trial -and- error elimination diet. This automatically eliminates many hazards and foods. The patient should keep to organic, untreated, unprocessed foods as far as possible and should do away with another set of hazards such as pesticides, various sprays and other poisons.

After having eliminated as many disturbing factors as possible, a self-search should be carried out to ascertain any doubtful symptoms from foods. It is prudent to try a basic diet, not including suspected foods for two weeks until the cause is detected. The best way, though, to prevent or overcome allergies is to make stronger the overall physical resistance so as not to fall an easy prey to every allergen that comes along. To begin with, the patient should fast on fresh fruit juices for four or five days. Repeated short juice fasts are to be expected to result in better tolerance to previous allergies. Subsequent to the fruit juice fast, the patient can take a mono diet of vegetables or fruits such as carrots, grapes or apples, for one week. After that one more food is added to the mono diet. A week later the third food is added and so on. After four weeks, the protein foods can be introduced, one at a time.

In case an allergic reaction to a newly introduced food is noticed, it should be discontinued and a new food tried. In this way all real allergens can be sooner or later eliminated from the diet. The body requires a large alkaline reserve for its daily activity. The many emergencies of acid formation through the day from wrong foods, fatigue, mental stress and lack of sleep can be met by the competency of the alkaline reserves. Boosting the normal body reserve of alkaline by liberal use of alkaline- forming foods is necessary for those suffering from allergies.

The foods which should be barred from the diet are tea, cola drinks, alcohol, sugar, coffee, chocolate, sweets and foods containing sugar, tobacco, milk, cheese, butter, smoked, salted, refined cereals, meats, fish, chicken, pickled foods and foods containing any chemical additives, preservatives and flavouring. These foods cause either toxic accumulations or over stimulation of adrenal glands or strain on pancreatic enzymes production or disturb the blood sugar balance. For preventive purposes, the entire C complex vitamins - known as the bioflavonoid, are recommended. They slowly but surely strengthen cell permeability to help immunise the body from various allergies, in particular hay fever. Multiple allergies may result from poor adrenal gland functioning. In such cases liberal amounts of pantothenic acids help cure them, although the recuperation will take a number of weeks. An adequate intake of vitamin E is also advantageous as this vitamin possesses effective anti allergic properties, as some studies have shown.

For allergic conditions in which an element of stress is present, it is necessary to employ such methods as relaxation, exercise, meditation and mind control. These methods will lessen or remove stress and in so doing contribute towards the treatment of allergies. Yoga asanas like yogamudra, ardha matsyendrasana, sarvangasana, shavasana and anuloma viloma, pranayama are also beneficial.

Chapter 59

Venereal Diseases

Venereal diseases in naturopathy can be cured by natural remedy. Syphillis and gonorrhoea are quite agreeable to successful treatment by appropriate dietary and other natural methods, leaving no ill effects to mar the future life and happiness of their victims. The only harmless way of treating venereal disease is fasting. All cases of syphilis and gonorrhoea can be cured through the agency of the fast. This will not only thwart dreaded after effects, but will also to a great extent improve the whole general health level of the patient by a methodical cleansing of his system. The juice of an orange, in a glass of lukewarm water, may be taken during this period. If orange juice disagrees, vegetable juice may be taken. Each day while fasting, it should be ensured that the bowels are cleansed of the poisonous matter thrown off by the self cleansing process now set up by the body. This can be achieved through a tepid water enema. The fast may be continued from seven to fourteen days.

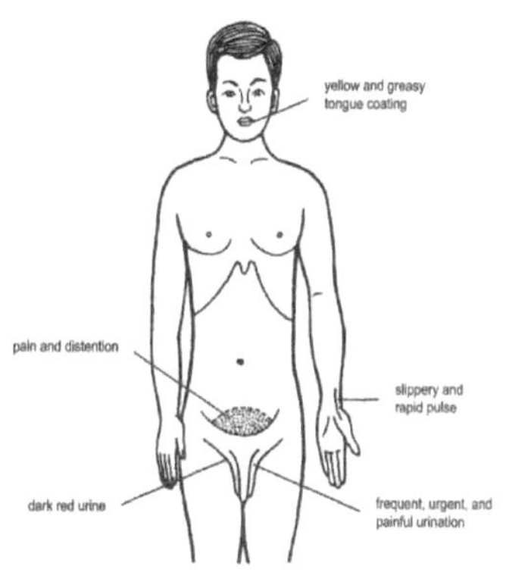

Subsequent to the fast, the patient may take on an exclusive fruit diet for further five days. He should consequently embark upon a balanced diet for three basic food groups namely seeds, nuts and grains, vegetables and fruits. Vegetable juices are extremely advantageous in the treatment of venereal diseases. Juices which are particularly helpful include those of carrot, cucumber, beet and spinach. The patient may make tolerant use of carrot juice either in combination with spinach juice or cucumber or beet. Amaranth (chaulai ka saag) is considered highly valuable in the treatment of Gonorrhoea. About twenty five grams of the leaves of this vegetable should be given twice or thrice a day to the patient in this condition.

Fresh juice of the flowers of the drumstick is very functional in the cure of gonorrhoea. For better results, this juice should be given twice on a daily basis with tender coconut water. It acts as a diuretic tonic medicine in this disease. A decoction of fresh lady`s fingers has also been found useful in treating gonorrhoea. A cupful of mucilage of lady`s finger is mixed with ripe banana and a glassful of buttermilk. The mixture is a very successful medication for Gonorrhoea. In case of syphilis, a `T` pack should be employed for an hour for the local treatment of the initial sore and it should be repeated twice on a daily basis. All clothes, sheets and towels, used by the patient should be handled cautiously to keep away from new sores and to prevent infection to others. It is better to boil all such articles. In case of eruptions on the different parts of the body, a wet sheet pack for an hour is beneficial. It will help bring out all the poisonous substances of the skin by producing more eruptions which will slowly but surely dry up.

Application of pelvic packs occasionally for an hour is one of the most useful methods of treatment in case of gonorrhoea. As irritation in the prostate gland and urethra is present in this disease, a hot hip bath for eight minutes has a valuable effect as it tends to reduce irritation. An occasional steam bath for eight minutes is of excellent value in both syphilis and gonorrhoea. It will help to get rid of the poisonous substances from the body and facilitate the kidney to execute its work efficiently. An overall massage has also advantageous effects on the entire body.

Chapter 60

Pleurisy

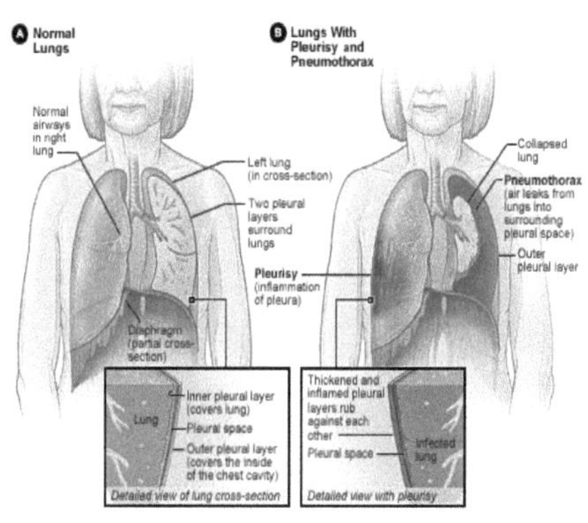

Natural remedy for pleurisy requires that the patient should observe a complete fast, abstaining from all liquid and solid foods. Nothing should be taken apart from plain water, hot or cold, as desired. Water may have bad taste, but at least three or four glasses should be taken on a daily basis for the first few days. The quantity of water should be steadily increased to five or six or more glasses each day. It would be helpful if during this period of fasting, a full warm enema is also taken once on a daily basis. A hot chest pack should be applied two or three times a day allowing it to remain for an hour or so each time. If the fever becomes high, the packs may be changed to cold ones. If, however, the reaction is not prompt and complete, it would be wise to use the hot packs.

Heat is always helpful for relieving the sharp pain coupled with pleurisy. This should be applied for half an hour twice on a daily basis. The patient should carry out deep breathing during this period. Sufficient rest and abundance of fresh air are vital.

In cases of dry pleurisy, further respite from pain can be obtained by strapping the chest. Heat is not used when the tapping is employed. A neutral immersion bath at 100 degree F for one hour on a daily basis has also been found advantageous in the treatment of pleurisy. After the acute symptoms have subsided, the patient may take on a milk diet. In this course of therapy, he should take 250 ml. of milk every two hours on the first day, every one and half hour on the second day, every hour on the third day and every three-quarters of an hour on the fourth day and onwards.

After the patient has gained slightly in strength, he should embark on moderate exercise as a routine, avoiding exhaustion. Air bath, sun bath and dry friction bath are of particular importance. If there is any particular disease, present along with the pleurisy whether as a causative or as a complicating condition, the same should also be given proper attention. Chronic pleurisy should be treated in the same manner as to the diet and the application of heat. All efforts should be made to boost the vitality, lessen toaxemia, and reinstate normal freedom of chest movements. A number of short fasts, at regular intervals, followed by milk diet may be required depending on the improvement for complete resurgence.

Chapter 61

Halitosis

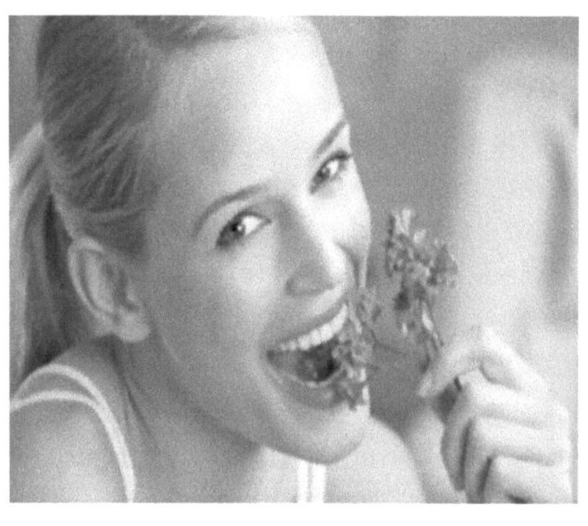

In the natural remedy for the treatment of halitosis, first and foremost the causes must be treated. If halitosis is caused by tooth and gum conditions, tonsillitis, sinusitis, smoking or anaemia, these conditions must be treated. Once they are eliminated the bad breath will wane. In the same way, bad breath resulting from gastrointestinal disorders can be successfully treated by correcting these disorders and cleansing the system of morbid matter. The patients suffering from halitosis should take a well balanced diet consisting of seeds, nuts and grains, vegetables and fruits, with emphasis on raw and cooked vegetables and fruits.

In case of constipation, all measures should be adopted for its eradication. The patient should stay away from carbohydrate foods, such as white sugar, white bread and products made from them as well as flesh foods and egg. Even whole grain bread should be eaten in moderation. The patient should also keep away from over eating of any kind of foods. He should eat six to eight soaked prunes and a few dried and soaked figs with breakfast. He must also drink the water in which these fruits were soaked. He should take plenty of liquids and drink six to eight glasses of water on a daily basis. This will help to eliminate bad breath. The teeth should be cleaned on a regular basis twice a day particularly before going to bed at night. Metal particles should be removed cautiously with toothpicks. In case of decaying teeth and swollen and bleeding gums, a dentist should be consulted. Munching a raw apple or guava after lunch removes most of the trapped particles.

The use of twigs of the margosa or neem tree as toothbrush is the best technique of cleaning the teeth.

Among the number of home remedies for halitosis, the use of fenugreek (methi) has proved most successful. A tea made from the seeds of the vegetables should be taken on a regular basis for correcting the condition. This tea is prepared by putting a teaspoon of seeds in half a litre of cold water and allowing it to simmer for fifteen minutes over a low flame. It should then be strained and used as tea. One more effective medication for bad breath is the use of avocodo (kulu naspati) which is far greater to any mouth lotion or remedies for this condition. It efficiently removes intestinal putrefaction or decomposition which is one of the most important causes of bad breath. The unripe guava (amrud) is functional in halitosis. It is rich in tannic, malic, oxalic and phosphoric acids as well as calcium, oxalate and manganese. Chewing it is a superb tonic for the teeth and gums. It helps cure bleeding from gums due to stypic effect and stops bad breath. Chewing tender leaves of guava tree also stops bleeding from gums and bad breath.

Parsley (prajmoda) is valuable in the treatment of bad breath. Two cups of water should be boiled and several springs of parsley, thickly chopped, should be stepped in this water along with two or three whole cloves or a quarter spoons of ground cloves. This mixture should be stirred occasionally while cooling. It should then be strained and used as a mouth wash and gargled more than a few times a day. All fruit and vegetable juices are advantageous in the treatment of halitosis and should be taken generously by those suffering from this disorder. Juices from fruits like apple, grape-fruit, (chakatora), lemon and pineapple, and vegetables like tomato, carrot and celery are in particular beneficial. The person suffering from bad breath should take plenty of exercise as lack of adequate exercise is one of the main causes of constipation leading to halitosis.

Chapter 62

Intestinal Worms

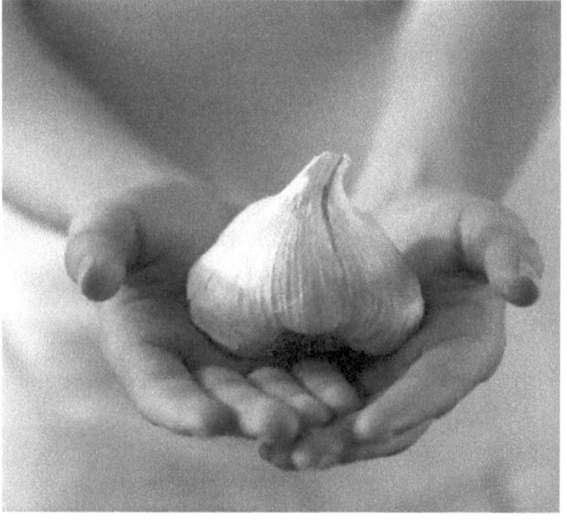

Natural remedy for intestinal worms should start on with diet. The patient should be kept on an exclusive diet of fresh fruits for five to seven days. Subsequently he may take on a well balanced light diet consisting mainly of fruits, vegetables, milk and whole meal bread. The diet should keep out fatty foods such as butter, cream, and oil, refined foods and all flesh foods. This dietary should be continued till the parasites are totally eliminated. In some cases, depending on the improvement being made, the all fruit diet may have to be repeated at regular intervals. In persistent cases the patient should resort to short fasts on raw fruit and vegetable juices. This fast has to be of a comparatively long duration in case of tapeworms. It would be prudent to carry on this fast treatment under the supervision of a naturopath, or better still, in a nature cure hospital. At the time of the all fruit diet or fasting period, the bowels should be cleansed on a daily basis with the tepid water enema.

Amongst the numerous home remedies found advantageous in the treatment of intestinal worms, the use of coconut is most successful. It is an ancient therapy for expelling all kinds of intestinal worms. A tablespoon of the freshly ground coconut should be taken at breakfast followed by a dose of castor oil after three hours. The procedure may be repeated till the treatment is complete. Garlic has been used for expelling intestinal worms from ancient times by the Chinese, Greeks, Romans, Hindus and Babylonians. It is also used by modern biological practitioners for this reason. Both fresh garlic and its oil are effective. An ancient technique of its medication was to place a couple of cloves of fresh garlic in its shoe. As the person walks, it is crushed and the worm killing garlic oil is absorbed by the skin and carried by blood into the intestines as it possesses the powerful penetrative force. This method is worth a trial by those who do not like the taste of garlic and cannot eat it.

The carrot is valuable in the elimination of threadworms from children as it is offensive to all parasites. A small cup of grated carrot taken every morning, with no other food added to the meal, can clear these worms rapidly. The digestive enzyme papain in the milk juice of the unripe papaya is a potent anthelmintic for destroying roundworms. Papaya seeds are also functional for this purpose. They are rich in a substance called caricin which is a very useful medicine for expelling roundworms. The alkaloid Carpaine found in the leaves has also the power to destroy or expel intestinal worms. They are given with honey. The bark, both of the root and the stems of pomegranate (anar) tree, is well known for its anthelmintic properties of destroying parasitic worms. The root-bark is, however, preferred as it contains larger quantity of the alkaloid punicine than the stem bark. This alkaloid is extremely toxic to tapeworms.

The seeds of the ripe pumpkin are useful in intestinal worms, in particular tapeworms. A mixture, prepared from the seeds after they are peeled and crushed, will kill parasites and help in expelling the tapeworm. It will be essential to fast for a day and empty the intestines by taking the juice of boiled dry prunes. The next day, three or four tumblers of this pumpkin seed infusion should be taken.

Chapter 63

Cholera

NATURAL-HOMEREMEDIES
Boil guava leaf in water &
drink that mixture

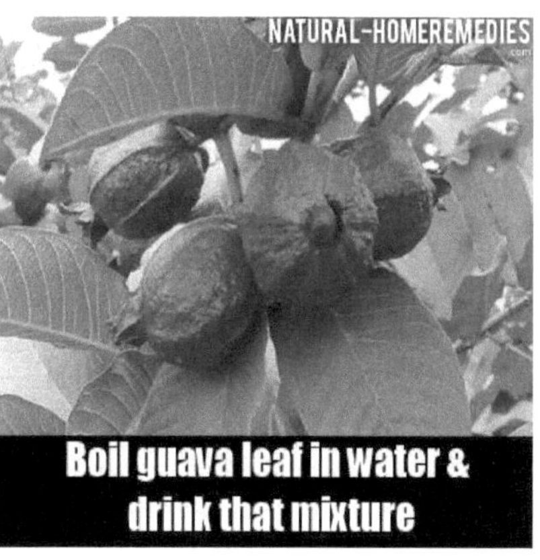

Natural remedy for cholera should in the beginning aim at fighting the loss of fluids and salts from the body. To relieve thirst, water, soda water or green coconut water should be given for sipping although this may be thrown out by vomiting. As a result, only small quantities of water should be given over and over again, as these may remain for sometime within the stomach and stay of every one minute means some absorption. This will moderate internal temperature and check the propensity to vomit. Intravenous infusions of saline solution should be given to reimburse for the loss of fluids and salts from the body. The patient may require five litres or more a day. Care should, however, be taken to avoid water logging the patient. Potassium may be added to the infused fluid. Rectal saline may sometimes prove functional for adults. Normally, half a litre of saline, with thirty grams of glucose, should be given per rectum every four hours until urine is passed freely.

After the acute stage of cholera is over, the patient may be given green coconut water and barley water in very thin form. When the stools begin to form, he should be given butter-milk. As he progresses towards recuperation, rice softened to semi-solid form mixed with curd, may be given. The patient should not be given solid food till he has completely recovered. Liquid and plain foods, which the patient can consume without endangering a reoccurrence of the malady, are best. Lemon, onion, green chilies, vinegar and mint should be included in the daily diet during an epidemic of cholera.

Certain home remedies have been found advantageous in the cure of cholera. The foremost among these is the use of lemon. The juice of this fruit can kill cholera bacilli within a short time. It is also a very efficient and dependable preventive food item against cholera during the epidemic. It can be taken in the form of sweetened or salted beverages for this purpose. Taking of lemon with food as daily routine can also thwart cholera. The root bark of guava is another valuable remedy. It is rich in tannins and can be effectively employed in the form of concentrated decoction in cholera. It will arrest vomiting and symptoms of Diarrhoea.

Onion is very helpful in cholera. About thirty grams of this vegetable and seven black peppers should be delicately pounded in a pestle and given to the patient. It allays thirst and restlessness and the patient feels better. The fresh juice of bitter gourd or karela is one more effective medicine in the early stages of cholera. Two teaspoons of this juice, mixed with an equal quantity of white onion juice and a teaspoon of lime juice, should be given Cholera can be controlled only by rigid purification of water supplies and proper disposal of human wastes. In case of the slightest uncertainty about the contamination of the water, it must be boiled before use, for drinking and cooking purposes. All foodstuffs must be kept covered and vegetables and fruits washed with a solution of potassium permanganate before consumption.

Other precautions against this disease comprise avoiding all uncooked vegetables, thorough washing of hands by all those who handle food, and elimination of all contacts with the disease.

Chapter 64

Cancer

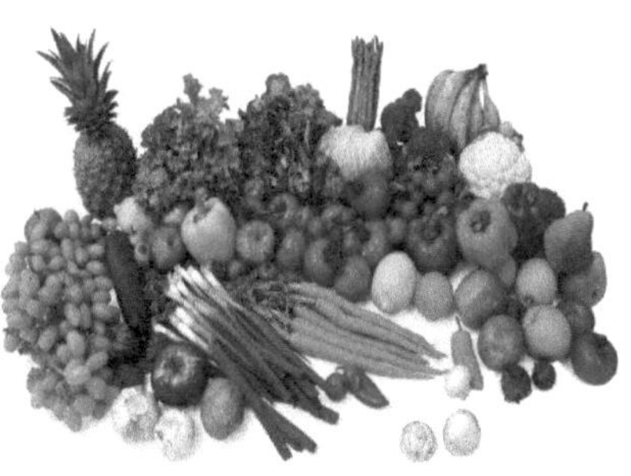

Naturopathy offers a natural remedy to cancer which comprises a complete change in diet, besides total elimination of all environmental sources of carcinogens, such as smoking and carcinogenic chemicals in air, water and food. The disease can be prevented and even treated by dietary programmes that include `natural foods `and the use of megavitamin supplements. As a first step, the patient should cleanse the system by thoroughly relieving constipation and making all the organs of elimination the skin, lungs, liver, kidneys and bowels active. Enemas should be used to cleanse the colon. For the first four or five days, the patient should consume only juicy fruits like oranges, grapefruits, lemons, apples, peaches, pears, pineapples and tomatoes. Vegetable juices are also useful, in particular carrot juice.

After a few days of an exclusive fruit diet, the patient may be given a nourishing alkaline-based diet. It should consist of 100 per cent natural foods, with emphasis on raw fruits and vegetables, particularly carrots, green leafy vegetables, cabbage, onion, garlic, cucumber, asparagus, beets and tomatoes. Almonds, millet, sesame seeds, sprouted seeds and grains, may also be added to the diet. Grape diet is an effective treatment of cancer.

After a short fast, the patient should have a grape meat every two hours from 8 a.m. to 8 p.m. This should be followed for a week or two even a month or two, in chronic cases of long standing. The patient should begin the grape cure with a small quantity of 30, 60, to 90 grams per meal, gradually increasing this to double the quantity. In course of time, about 250 grams may safely be taken as a meal.

Recent researches have shown that certain vitamins can be effectively employed in the fight against cancer and that they can increase the life expectancy of some incurable cancer patients. A mixture of vitamin C and copper compound has lethal effects on cancer. According to several studies, vitamin A exerts an inhibiting effect on carcinogenesis. It is one of the most important aids to the body's defence system to fight and prevent cancer. Recent studies from all over the world suggest that a liberal use of green and yellow vegetables and fruits can prevent cancer.

Chapter 65

Colitis

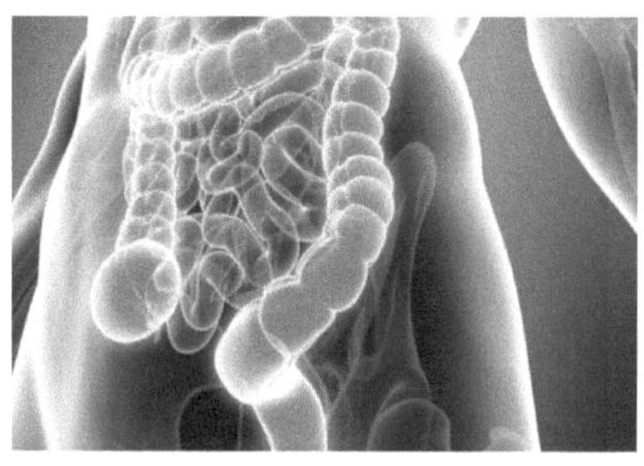

Naturopathy offers a natural cure for colitis. In the natural remedy, diet plays an important part in the treatment. At the initial stage, plain warm water with a little olive oil is consumed which is the only method of softening and removing the accumulations of hardened matter sticking to the walls of the colon. It is wise to observe a juice fast for five days or so in most cases of ulcerative colitis. The juices may be diluted with a little boiled water. Papaya juice, raw cabbage and carrot juices will be in particular beneficial. Citrus juices should be avoided. The bowel should be cleansed daily with a warm water enema.

After the juice fast, the patient should gradually adopt a diet of small, regular meals of soft cooked or steamed vegetables, rice, dalia (coarsely broken wheat), well ripened fruits like banana and papaya, yogurt and home-made cottage cheese. Sprouted seeds and grains, whole meal bread and raw vegetables may be added gradually to this diet after about ten days. All food must be eaten slowly and chewed carefully. Foods which should be excluded from the diet are white sugar, white bread and white flour products, highly seasoned foods, highly salted foods, strong tea, coffee and alcoholic beverages and foods cooked in aluminium pans. Ripe bananas are highly advantageous in the treatment of ulcerative colitis, being bland, smooth, easily digested and slightly laxative.

Another valuable remedy for ulcerative colitis is the use of butter-milk. It is the residual milk left after the fat has been removed from yogurt by churning. Butter milk enema twice a week is also comforting and helps in re-installing a healthy flora in the colon. An effective cure for colitis is tender coconut water; it is soothing to the soft mucosa of the colon. Cooked apple also aids the healing of ulcerative conditions because of its sufficient concentration of iron and phosphorous. The patient should have a bowel movement at the same time each day and spend ten to fifteen minutes in the endeavour. Drinking two glasses of water the first thing in the morning will stimulate a normal bowel movement. An enema may be used if no bowel movement occurs. Complete bed rest and plenty of liquids are very essential. The patient should eliminate all causes of tension, adjust to his disability and face his anxiety with patience.

Chapter 66

Alcoholism

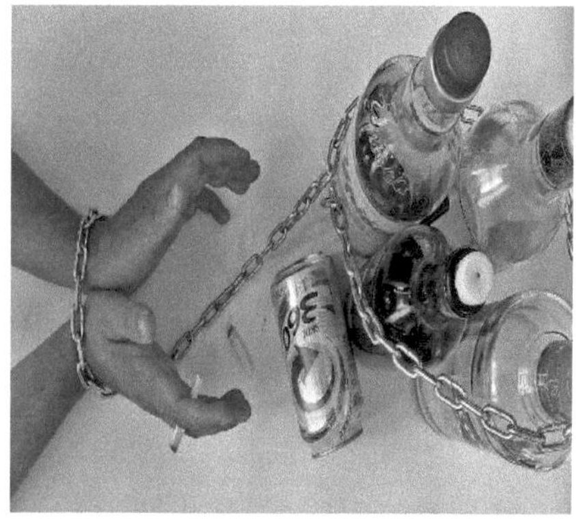

Alcoholism refers to addiction to alcohol and the natural remedy for alcoholism deals in building the body's nutritional integrity soaps to prevent craving for stimulants like drinks. Alcoholism is a chronic disorder, in which a person is unable to refrain from frequent and excess consumption of alcohol for physical or psychological reasons. Alcoholics have a puffy face with bloodshot eyes, a hoarse voice and a rapid pulse. Vomiting, delirium, impaired judgement and disturbed sleep are some of the other symptoms.

The chronic alcoholic first of all must make a firm resolution to stop drinking. He should abstain from alcohol all at once for the habit cannot be got rid of in gradual stages.

The most effective way to treat alcoholism is to build the body's nutritional integrity soaps to avert desire for stimulants like alcoholic drinks. The patients should be put on a cleansing juice fast for at least ten days in the beginning. During this period, he should have juice of an orange every two hours from 8 a.m. to 8 p.m. If orange juice does not agree, vegetable juices may be taken. Each day while fasting, bowels should be cleansed of effete and poisonous matter thrown off by the self-cleansing process set up by the body. This can be achieved by warm water enema.

After the preliminary fast on juices, the most favourable diet of vital nutrients is essential. Such a diet should consist of whole grains, cereals, nuts, seeds and sprouts, fresh fruits and vegetables. It is advisable that in the beginning of the treatment, the patient is given a suitable substitute to relieve the craving if and when such a craving occurs. The best substitute drink for alcohol is a glass of fresh fruit juice, sweetened with honey, if desired. In the alternative, wholesome candy may be taken. The patient should always have easily available juices, candy, or other snacks to be taken between meals if he feels a craving for a stimulant.

All refined foods such as sugar, white rice, macaroni products and white flour and meat should be avoided. The patient should eat several small meals a day in preference to two or three large ones and avoid strong condiments such as pepper, mustard, and chilli. He should not smoke as this will only increase his desire for alcohol. Apples are considered valuable in the treatment of alcoholism as their use removes intoxication and reduces the desire for wine and other intoxicating liquors. The raw celery juice is also considered helpful. It has a sobering effect and is an antidote to alcohol. In addition to proper nutrition, plenty of rest and outdoor exercises are necessary. The healthy condition of the appetite center, which controls the craving for alcohol, is improved by exercise. Yoga asanas for general health such as padmasana, vajrasana, vakrasana, paschimottanasana, yogamudra, bhujangasana, halasana and salabhasana will be beneficial. Copious drinking of water, hot fomentations on the stomach and abdomen with a wet girdle pack between applications are also effective water treatment for alcoholism.

Chapter 67

Arteriosclerosis

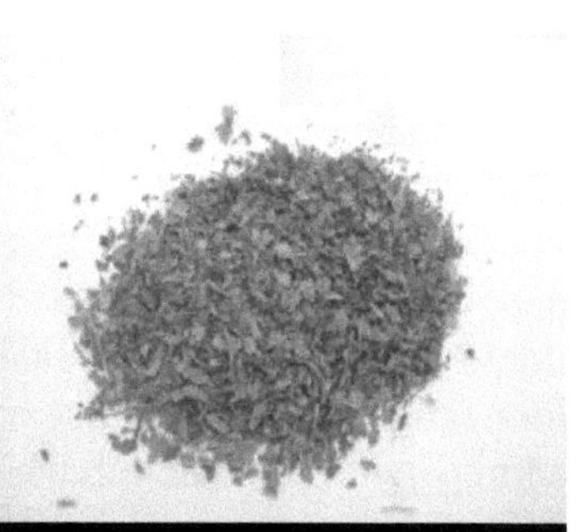

Boil a cup of water and mix dry parsley with it and appy to treat Arteriosclerosis

Natural remedy for arteriosclerosis involves resorting to a short juice fast for five to seven days. If the causes of arteriosclerosis are known, remedial action should be taken promptly to remove them. All available fresh, raw vegetables and fruit juices in season may be consumed. Grape-fruit juice, pineapple juice, lemon juice and juices of green vegetables are particularly beneficial. A warm water enema should be used daily to cleanse the bowels during the period of fasting. After the juice fast, the patient should take optimum diet made up from three basic food groups, namely (i) seeds, nuts and grains, (ii) vegetables and, (iii) fruits, with emphasis on raw foods.

Cold pressed vegetable oils, particularly safflower oil, flax seed oil and olive oil should be used on a regular basis. Further, shorter fasts on juices may be undertaken at intervals of three months or so, depending on the improvement. The patient should take a number of small meals instead of a few large ones. The patient should avoid all hydrogenated fats and a surplus of saturated fats, such as butter, cream, ghee and animal fat. He should also avoid meat, salt and all refined and processed foods, condiments, sauces, pickles , strong tea, coffee, white sugar, white flour and all products made from them. Foods cooked in aluminium and copper utensils should not be taken as toxic metals entering the body are known to be deposited on the walls of the aorta and the arteries.

Smoking, if habitual, should be given up if someone suffers from arteriosclerosis as smoking constricts the arteries and aggravates the condition. Recent investigations have shown that garlic and onions have a preventive effect on the development of arteriosclerosis.

Vitamin C has also proved valuable as it helps in the conversion of cholesterol into bile acids. One of the most useful home remedies for arteriosclerosis is the lemon peel. It is believed to be one of the richest known sources of vitamin P. It strengthens the entire arterial system. Shredded lemon peel may be added to soups and stews or sprinkled over salads.

Parsley is another effective home cure for arteriosclerosis. It contains element which help to maintain the blood vessels, mainly the capillaries and arterial system in a healthy condition. It may be taken as a beverage by simmering it gently in the water for a few minutes and partaking several times daily. The beet juice has also proved valuable in arteriosclerosis. It is an excellent solvent for inorganic calcium deposit. Juices of carrot and spinach are also advantageous. These juices can be taken individually or in combination. Prolonged neutral immersion baths at bed time on alternate days is beneficial. This bath is administered in a bath tub which should be properly fitted with hot and cold water connection.

Chapter 68

Backache

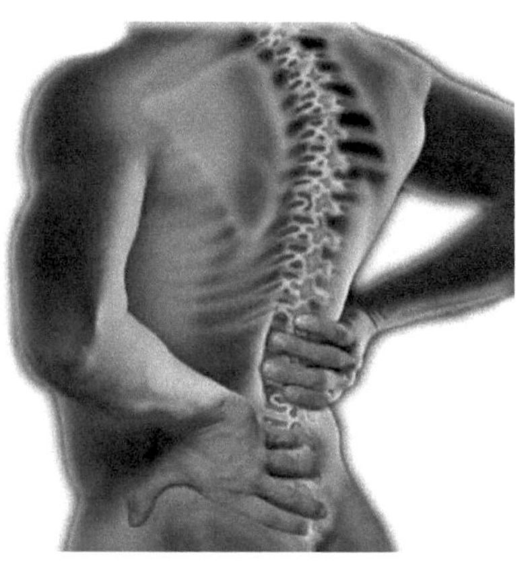

Natural remedy for backache in naturopathy is exercise which improves the supply of nutrients to spinal discs, thereby delaying the process of deterioration that comes with age. Naturopathy offers a number of natural remedy to relieve and prevent backache.

Exercise is considered to be the most effective natural cure for backache. Exercise helps to improve the supply of nutrients to spinal discs, thereby delaying the process of deterioration that comes with age. Safe exercises include walking, swimming and bicycling. Controlling one`s weight is another important step towards relieving backache as excess weight greatly increases the stress on soft back tissues.

Yoga asanas which are beneficial in the treatment of backache are bhujangasana, salabhasana, halasana, uttanapadasana and shavasana. The back can be strengthened through proper nutrition, exercise and relaxation and in the process general health will also improve.

Those with sedentary occupations should take a break to stand up every hour. Soft cushioned seats should be avoided and position should be changed as often as possible. Persons with back problems should sleep on a firm mattress on their sides with knees bent at right angles to the torso. They should take care never to bend from the waist down to lift any object but instead should swat close to the object, bending the knees but keeping the back straight, and then stand up slowly. Neck tension arising from long hours at the desk or behind the wheel of the car can be relieved by certain neck exercises. These include rotating the head clockwise and anticlockwise, allowing the head to drop forward and backward as far as possible and turning the head to the right and left as far as possible several times. These exercises help to loosen up contracted neck muscles which may restrict the blood supply to the head.

The diet of those suffering from backache should consist of a salad of raw vegetables such as tomato, carrot, cabbage, cucumber, radish, lettuce and at least two steamed or lightly cooked vegetables such as cauliflower, cabbage, carrot, spinach and plenty of fruits, all except bananas. The patients should have four meals daily. They may take fruits and milk during breakfast, steamed vegetables and whole wheat chapattis during lunch, fresh fruits or fruit juice in the evening and a bowl of raw salad and sprouts during dinner. The patients should avoid fatty, spicy, and fried foods, curd, sweetmeats, sugar, condiments as well as tea and coffee. Those who smoke and take tobacco in any form should give them up completely.

Proteins and vitamin C are essential for the development of healthy bone. Vitamin D, calcium, phosphorous and the essential minerals are vital for healthy bones. Foods that have been processed for storage to avoid spoiling have few nutrients and should be eliminated from the diet. Vitamin C has proved helpful in relieving low-back pain and averting spinal disc operations. Hot fomentations, alternate sponging or application of radiant heat to the back will also give instant relief.

Chapter 69

Defective Vision

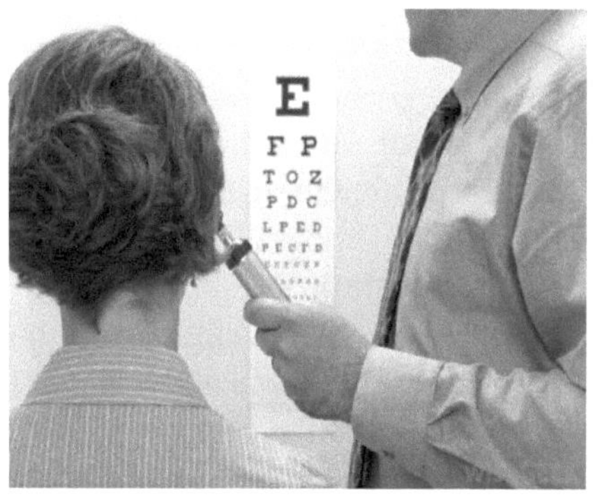

Exercise is the most important natural remedy for defective vision. In case of eye exercise the patient should keep his head still and relaxed. The eyes should be gently moved up and down. The movement is to be repeated twice or thrice at two seconds intervals. The eyes should be moved from side to side as far as possible, without any force or effort six times. Another eye exercise is to hold the index finger of the right hand about eight inches in front of the eyes and then look from the finger to any other large object ten or more feet away. This exercise should be done fairly rapidly.

In neck exercises the neck should be rotated in circles and semi circles. The shoulders should be moved clockwise and anti-clockwise briskly, drawing them up as far as possible several times. The head should be allowed to draw forward and backward as far as possible. These exercises help to loosen up contracted neck muscles which may restrict blood supply to the head. Sun gazing also helps to cure defective vision. The patient should sit on a bench facing the sun with your eyes closed and gently sway sideways several times for eighteen minutes. He should open the eyes and blink about ten times at the sun and look at some greenery. This helps short sight and is good for inflamed eyes. Splashing plain, cold water several times on closed eyes cools the eyes and boosts blood supply.

Swinging is also an effective exercise in curing vision. The patient should stand on his feet twelve inches apart with hands held loosely at the sides, the whole body and mind relaxed. Gently he should sway his body from side to side, slowly, steadily, with the heels rising alternatively but not the rest of the foot. Swinging should be done in front of a window or a picture. When the patient faces one end of the window or object, he should blink once. This exercise has a very beneficial effect upon the eyes and nervous system. Diet therapy is an essential part in the treatment of defective vision. Natural, uncooked foods are the best diet. These include fresh fruits, such as oranges, apples, grapes, peaches, plums and cherries. Green vegetable like lettuce, cabbage, spinach, turnip tops; root vegetables like potatoes, turnips, carrot, onions and beetroots; nuts, dried fruits and dairy products are also useful.

Cereals are also necessary, but they should only be consumed sparingly. Genuine whole meal bread is the best and most suitable. The value of vitamin A for improving vision must be stressed. The intake of sufficient quantities of this vitamin is essential as a safeguard against or treatment of defective vision or eye disease of any kind. The best sources of this vitamin are cod liver oil, raw spinach, turnip tops, cream, cheese, butter, egg yolk, tomatoes, lettuce, carrot, cabbage, soya beans, green peas, wheat germ, fresh milk, oranges and dates. Certain yoga asanas such as bhujangasana, salabhasana, yogamudra, paschimottanasana and kriyas like jalneti are also beneficial for the eyes.

Chapter 70

Diarrhoea

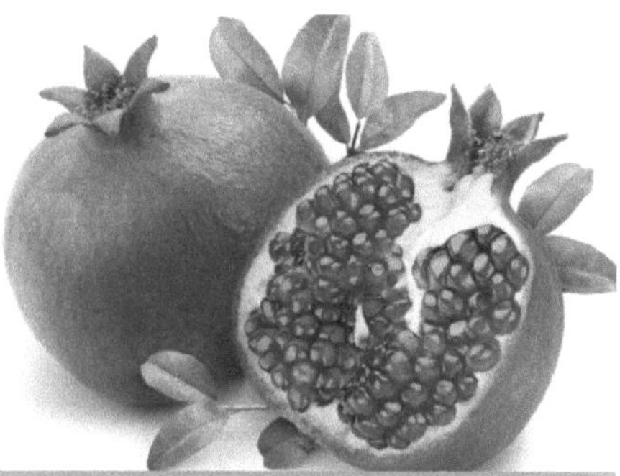

Pomegranate Juice For Diarrhea

In the natural remedy for diarrhoea it is advisable that the patient keeps a complete fast for two days. Hot water only may be taken during the period to compensate for the loss of fluids. Juices of fruits may be taken after the severe symptoms are over. After the condition improves, meals can be enlarged steadily to include cooked vegetables, whole rice and milk. Raw foods should be taken only after the patient completely recovers. A successful remedy for Diarrhoea is the use of buttermilk. It is the residual milk left after the fat has been removed from yogurt by churning. It helps overcome injurious intestinal flora and re-establish the friendly flora. The acid in the buttermilk also fights germs and bacteria. It may be taken and mixed with a pinch of salt three or four times a day controlling Diarrhoea.

Carrot soup is another effective home medication for diarrhoea. It supplies water to fight dehydration, replenishes sodium, potassium, phosphorus, calcium, and magnesium, supplies pectin and coats the intestine to allay inflammation. It checks the expansion of harmful intestinal bacteria and prevents vomiting. The pomegranate has proved beneficial in the treatment of Diarrhoea on account of its astringent properties. Mango seeds are also helpful in Diarrhoea. The seeds should be collected during the mango season, dried in the shade and powdered and kept stored for use as medicine when required. Turmeric is another effective home remedy for Diarrhoea. It is a very useful intestinal antiseptic. It is also a gastric stimulant and a tonic. Turmeric rhizome, its juice or dry powder are all very helpful in curing chronic diarrhoea.

In case of diarrhoea caused by indigestion, dry or fresh ginger is very useful. A piece of dry ginger is powdered along with a crystal or rock salt. A quarter teaspoonful of this powder should be taken with a small piece of jugglery. It will bring quick relief as ginger, being carminative, and aids digestion by stimulating the gastrointestinal tract. Starchy liquids such as arrowroot water, barley water, rice gruel and coconut water are highly beneficial in the treatment of diarrhoea. Other home remedies include bananas and garlic. Bananas contain pectin and encourage the growth of beneficial bacteria. Garlic is a powerful, effective and non-toxic antibiotic. It aids digestion and routs parasites.

Chapter 71

Fatigue

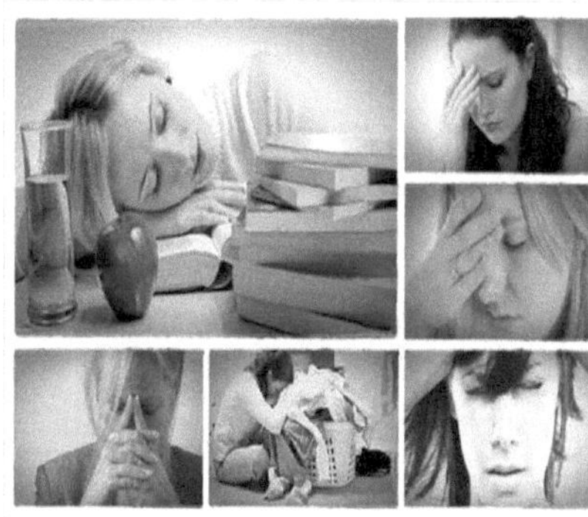

Nutritional measures are most essential in the natural treatment of fatigue. Proper eating habits are very important in the cure of fatigue. Studies reveal that people, who eat small mid-meals experience less from fatigue and nervousness, think more clearly and are well-organised than those who eat only three meals daily. These mid-meals should consist of fresh or dried fruits, fresh fruit or vegetable juices, raw vegetables or small sandwich of whole grain bread. The mid-meal should be small and less food should be consumed at regular meals. The patient should eat health foods which provide energy to the body.

The patient should take an optimum diet made up of (i) seeds, nuts and grains, (ii) vegetables, and (iii) fruits. Roughly, each food group should supply the bulk of one of the three meals. Sprouting is an exceptional way to eat seeds, beans and grains in raw form. Sprouting increases the nutritional value of foods and many new vitamins are created or multiplied in seeds during sprouting. The patient should supplement the three health building food groups with special protective foods such as milk, high quality cold-pressed unrefined vegetable oil and honey. The patient should also take natural vitamin and mineral supplements as an effective assurance against nutritional deficiencies, as such deficiencies have been found to be a factor in fatigue.

Lack of pantothenic acid, B vitamin in particular, leads to tremendous fatigue as deficiency of this vitamin is associated with tiredness of the adrenal glands. In fact the entire B-complex protects nerves and increases energy by helping to nurture and regulate glands. The vegetarian foods rich in vitamin B are wheat and other whole grain cereals, green leafy vegetables, rice polishing, milk, nuts, banana, yeast, pulses and peas. Minerals are also important. Potassium is particularly needed for protection against fatigue. Raw green vegetables are rich in this mineral. Calcium is indispensable for relaxation and is advantageous in cases of insomnia and tension both of which can lead to fatigue. Sodium and zinc are also beneficial in the treatment of fatigue.

Raw vegetable juices, especially carrot juice, taken separately or in combination with juices of beets and cucumbers are highly valuable in overcoming fatigue. The patient should avoid depending for an energy lift, on crutches such as taking aspirin, tranquilisers and other drugs, drinking coffee or alcohol, smoking, eating some sugar or sweets.

Chapter 72

Epilepsy

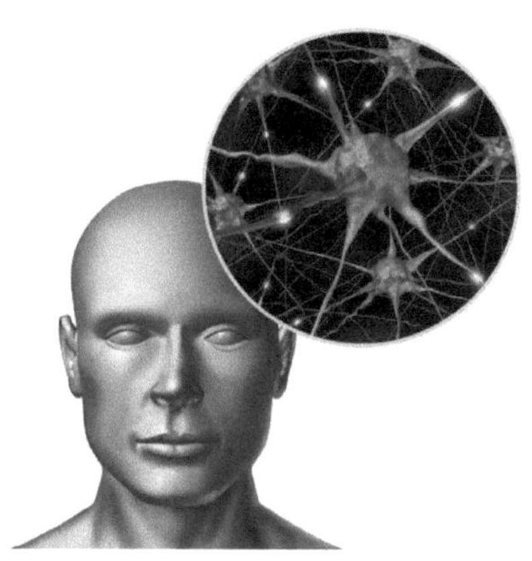

Natural remedy for epilepsy in naturopathy emphasises on cheerful living and healthy eating. It says that the patient must hold on to a simple and correct natural life. He must assume a cheerful, optimistic attitude; abstain from mental and physical overwork and worry.

The most important part of the treatment is the diet. To begin with, the patient should be placed on an exclusive fruit diet for first few days. During this period he should have three meals a day of fresh juicy fruits such as oranges, apples, grapes, grapefruit, peaches, pears, pineapple and melon. Thereafter, he may gradually adopt a well balanced diet of three basic food groups. The first group includes seeds, nuts and grains; the second group includes vegetables and the third group comprises of fruits with emphasis on sprouted seeds such as alfalfa seeds and raw vegetables and fruits.

The diet should consist of a modest amount of raw milk preferably goat's milk and milk products such as raw butter and homemade cottage cheese. The diet should eliminate completely all animal proteins, except milk, as they not only lack in magnesium, but also rob the body of its own magnesium storage as well as of vitamin B6. Both these substances are needed in large amounts by epileptics. The best food sources of magnesium are raw nuts, seeds, soyabeans, green leafy vegetables such as spinach, kale, beet-tops etc. The patient should avoid all refined foods, fried and greasy food, sugar and products made with it, strong tea, coffee, alcoholic beverages, condiments and pickles. The patient should avoid over eating and take frequent small meals rather than a few large ones.

Mud packs on the abdomen help to remove the toxaemic conditions of the intestines and thereby speed up elimination of epileptic conditions. The application of alternate hot and cold compresses to the base of the brain that is at the back of the head will be advantageous. The procedure is to dip the feet in a bucket of hot water and apply first a hot towel and then a cold one to the base of the brain. The alternate hot and cold towels should be kept for two or three minutes about four times. The process shall be repeated twice every day. Full Epsom-salt bath, twice a week are also beneficial. If the sufferer from epilepsy has taken strong drugs for many years, he should not leave off entirely all at once. The dosage may be cut to half to begin with and then gradually reduced further until it can be left off entirely.

An epileptic should firmly observe all the natural laws of good health and build and maintain the highest level of general health. He should remain active mentally but avoid all severe mental and physical stress. And above all, he should keep away from excitements of all kinds.

Chapter 73

Heart Disease

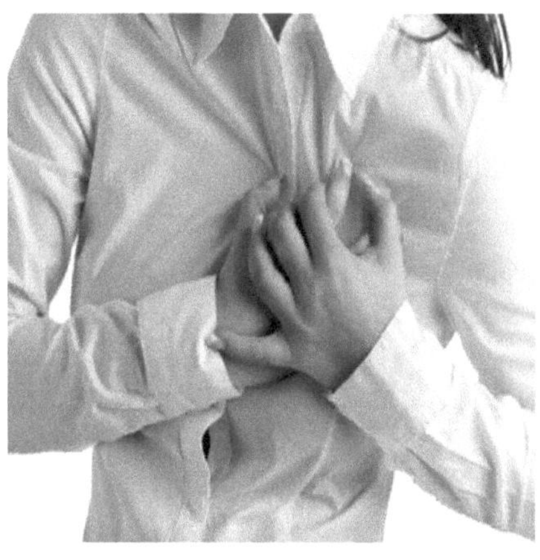

Natural remedy of heart disease in naturopathy is directed towards a well balanced diet. A curative diet designed to alter body chemistry and improve the quality of general nutritional intake can, in many cases, reverse the degenerative changes which have occurred in the heart and blood vessels. The diet should be lacto-vegetarian, low in sodium and calories. Foods which should be eliminated are all white flour products, sweets, chocolates, canned foods in syrup, soft drinks, squashes, all hard fats of animal origin such as butter, cream and fatty meats. Diet should incorporate high quality, natural organic foods, with emphasis on whole grains, seeds, fresh fruits and vegetables. Salt and sugar should be reduced considerably. The patient should also avoid tea, coffee, alcohol and tobacco.

A number of studies have indicated that garlic can reduce the cholesterol level in persons whose body in general cannot control the cholesterol fractions. Other important cholesterol lowering foods are alfalfa and yogurt. Best food sources are unrefined, raw, crude vegetable oils, seeds and grains. Fruits and vegetables in general are extremely beneficial in the cure of heart disease. Seasonal fruits are quite valuable heart tonics. Apples in particular contain heart stimulating properties and the patients suffering from the weakness of heart should make liberal use of apples and apple jams. Fresh grapes, pineapples, oranges, custard apples, pomegranates and coconut water also tone up the heart. Grapes are useful in heart pain and palpitation of the heart and the disease can be rapidly controlled if the patient adopts an exclusive grapes diet for few days. Grape juice in particular will be valuable when one is in fact suffering from a heart attack.

Indian gooseberry or amla is considered an effective home medication for heart disease. It tones up the functions of all the organs of the body and builds up health by destroying the heterogeneous elements and renewing lost energy. Another excellent home remedy for heart disease is onions. They are functional in normalising the percentage of blood cholesterol by oxidising excess cholesterol. One teaspoon of raw onion juice first thing in the morning will be extremely advantageous in such cases. Honey has marvellous properties to prevent all sorts of heart disease. It tones up the heart and improves the circulation. It is also effective in cardiac pain and palpitation of the heart. One tablespoonful on a daily basis after food is sufficient to prevent all sorts of heart troubles.

Patients afflicted with heart disease should increase their intake of foods rich in vitamin E, as this vitamin promotes the functioning of the heart by improving oxygeneration of the cells. Many whole meal products and green vegetables, particularly outer leaves of cabbage are good sources of vitamin E. The vitamin B group is vital for heart and circulatory disorders. The best sources of vitamin B are whole grains. Vitamin C is also important as it protects against spontaneous breaches in capillary walls which can lead to heart attacks. It also guards against high blood cholesterol. The stress of anger, fear, distress and similar emotions can raise blood fat and cholesterol levels instantly but this reaction to stress can do little harm if the diet is sufficient in vitamin C and pantothenic acid. The richest sources of vitamin C are citrus fruits.

The following is the suggested diet for persons suffering from hypertension or some disorder of the heart:

- **Breakfast:** Fresh fruit such as apples, grapes, pears, peaches, pineapple, orange, melons, one or two slices whole meal toast, yogurt, skimmed milk or soya milk.
- **Mid-morning:** Fresh fruit juice or coconut water.
- **Lunch:** Combination salad of vegetables such as lettuce, cabbage, endive, carrots, cucumber, beetroot, tomato, onion and garlic.
- **Mid-afternoon:** One or two whole meal biscuits and fruit juice.
- **Dinner:** Fresh fruit or vegetable juice or soup, two lightly cooked vegetables, one or two whole wheat tappets.

The patient should also pay attention to other laws of nature for health building such as taking moderate exercise, getting proper rest and sleep, adopting the right mental attitude and getting fresh air and drinking pure water.

The use of an ice bag on the spinal area between the second and tenth thoracic vertebrae for thirty minutes three times a week, a hot compress applied to the left side of the neck for thirty minutes every alternate day and massage of the abdomen and upper back muscles are water treatments which are beneficial in cases of heart disease. Hot foot and hand baths are exceptional for relieving the pain of angina pectoris. Asanas such as shavasana, vajrasana, and gomukhasna, yogic kriyas like jalneti and pranayamas such as shitali, sitkari and bhramari are also helpful in providing respite to heart patients.

Chapter 74

Indigestion

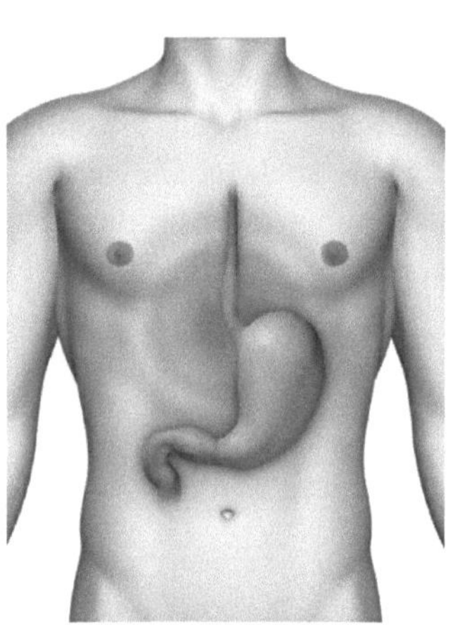

In naturopathy the best way to commence the treatment for indigestion is to adopt an all-fruit diet for about five days. After the all-fruit diet, the patient may take to a restricted diet of easily digestible foods, consisting of lightly cooked vegetables, juicy fruits and buttermilk for about ten days. He may subsequently embark upon a well balanced diet. The use of fruits in general is advantageous in the treatment of indigestion. They flush out the undigested food reside and restore health to perfect order. Being rich in water, they clean body mechanisms thoroughly. The best among the fruits in dyspepsia is lemon. Its juice reaches the stomach and attacks the bacteria, inhabiting the formation of acids. Lemon juice removes indigestion by dislodging this acid and other harmful substances from the stomach, thereby strengthening and prompting a healthy appetite.

The orange is another valuable food remedy in chronic indigestion. It stimulates the flow of digestive juices thereby improving digestion and increasing appetite. It creates appropriate conditions for the development of friendly bacteria in the intestines. Another fruit useful in indigestion is grapes. They are a light food which removes indigestion and irritation of the stomach in a short time and relieves heat. Pineapple is also valuable. It acts as a tonic in dyspepsia and relieves much of the digestives disorders of dyspeptics. Half a glass of pineapple juice should be taken after a meal in this condition.

The sufferer from indigestion should never eat and drink together. Water or other liquids should be taken half an hour before and one hour after a meal. Milk, buttermilk and vegetables soups are, however, foods and can be taken with meals. The patient of indigestion should eat very slowly and chew food as thoroughly as possible. Food should not be taken if appetite is lacking. A meal or two can be missed if necessary, until real appetite returns. Vegetables should never be boiled but steamed. Eating raw vegetables and raw fruits should be avoided.

Yogic asanas such as ardh-matsyasana, sarvangasana, uttanapadasana, pavana muktasana, vajrasana, yogamudra, bhujangasana, salabhasana, and shavasana, kriyas like jalneti and kunjal, and pranayamas like kapalbhati, anuloma-viloma, and ujjai are extremely helpful in the treatment of indigestion. Light exercises such as walking, golf and swimming also help digestion. A daily enema should be administered to cleanse toxic bowel waste. Other beneficial water treatments include wet girdle pack applied at night, application of ice bags over the stomach half an hour after meals, a daily cold friction bath and alternate hot and cold hip baths at night. Massaging of the abdomen also helps in the cure of indigestion.

Chapter 75

Kidney Stones

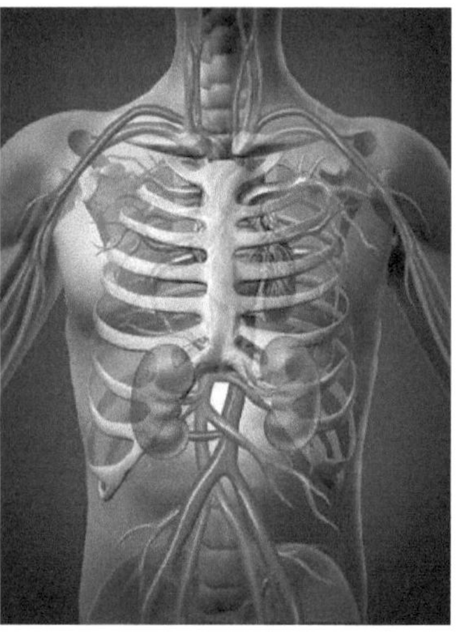

In the natural remedy of kidney stones the patient should avoid foods which irritate the kidneys, to control acidity or alkalinity of the urine and to ensure adequate intake of fluids to prevent the urine from becoming concentrated. The foods considered irritants to the kidneys are alcoholic beverages, condiments, pickles, certain vegetables like cucumbers, tomatoes, spinach, rhubarb, water-cress and those with strong aroma such as asparagus, onions, beans, cabbage and cauliflower, meat, gravies and carbonated waters.

For controlling the formation of calcium phosphate stones, a moderately low calcium and phosphorous diet should be taken. The intake of calcium and phosphates should be restricted to minimal levels consistent with maintaining nutritional adequacy. In this diet, milk should constitute the main source of calcium and curd or cottage cheese, lentils and groundnuts should form the main sources of phosphorous. Foods which should be avoided are whole wheat flour, Bengal gram, peas, soyabeans, beets, spinach, cauliflower, turnips, carrots, almonds and coconuts.

When stones are composed of calcium and magnesium phosphates and carbonates, the diet should be so regulated as to maintain acidic urine. In such a diet, only half a liter of milk, two servings of fruits and two servings of vegetables should be taken. The vegetables may consist of asparagus, fresh green peas, squash, pumpkins, turnips, cauliflower, cabbage and tomatoes. For fruits, watermelon, grapes, peaches, pears, pineapple, papayas and guavas may be taken. When the stones contain oxalate, foods with high oxalic acid content should be avoided. These foods include almonds, beetroots, brinjal, brown bread, cabbage, cherry, and chocolate, French Beans, potatoes, radish, spinach and soyabeans. Uric stones occur in patients who have an increased uric acid in the blood and increased uric acid exertion in the urine. Kidney beans, also known as French beans or common beans, are regarded as a very effective remedy for kidney problems, including kidney stones.

In case of kidney stones, basil juice and honey should be taken for six months. It has been found that the stones can be expelled from the urinary tract with this treatment. The celery is also a valuable food for those who are prone to stone formation in the kidneys or the gall bladder. Its regular use prevents future tone formation. Research has shown the remarkable therapeutic success of vitamin B6 or pyridoxine in the treatment of kidney stones. This treatment has to be continued for several months for obtaining a permanent cure. Certain yoga asanas such as pavana-muktasana, uttanpadasana, bhujangasana, dhanursana and halasana are also highly beneficial as they stimulate the kidneys.

Chapter 76

Obesity

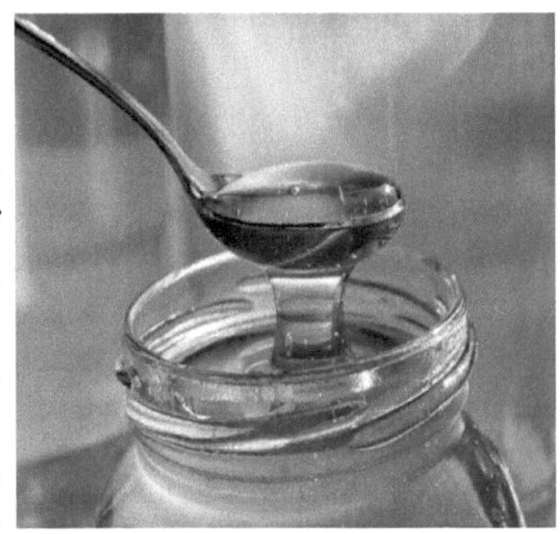

In natural remedy of obesity, the chief concern should be the balanced selection of foods which supply the maximum necessary nutrients with the least number of calories. Exercise also forms an important part of the treatment. To begin with, patient should undertake a juice fast for seven to ten days. Juices of lemon, grape fruit, orange, pineapple, cabbage, celery, may be taken during this period. Long juice fast up to forty days can also be undertaken, but only under expert guidance and supervision. After the juice fast, the patient should spend a further four or five days on an all-fruit diet, taking three meals of fresh juicy fruits such as oranges, grapefruit, pineapple and papaya. Subsequently, he may steadily embark upon a low-calorie well balanced diet of three basic food groups, namely (i) seeds, nuts and grains, (ii) vegetables and (iii) fruits, with emphasis on raw fruits, vegetables, and fresh juices.

The foods which should be radically curtailed or altogether avoided are high-fat foods such as butter, cheese, chocolates, ice-cream, fat meats, fried foods, and gravies. High carbohydrate foods like bread, candy, cake, cookies, cereal products, legumes, potatoes, honey, sugar, syrup and rich puddings beverages such as all-fountain drinks and alcoholic drinks should also be avoided. Fasting on honey -lime juice water is extremely beneficial in the cure of obesity without the loss of energy and appetite. In this mode of treatment, one spoon of fresh honey should be mixed with a juice of half a lime in a glass of lukewarm water and taken at on a regular basis.

Another effective therapy for obesity is a restricted lemon juice diet. On the first day the patient should be given nothing but ample of water. On the second day juice of three lemons mixed with equal amount of water should be given. One lemon should be subsequently increased each day until the juice of twelve lemons is consumed per day. Then the number of lemons should be decreased in the same order until three lemons are taken in a day. The patient may feel weak and hungry on the first two days, but afterwards the condition will be stabilised by itself. Cabbage is considered to be an effective home remedy for obesity.

Along with dietetic treatment, the patient should adopt all other natural methods of reducing weight. Exercise is an important part of weight reduction plan. It helps to use up calories stored in body fat and relieves tension, besides toning up the muscles of the body. Certain yoga asana are highly beneficial. Not only do they break up or redistribute fatty deposits and help slimming, but they also strengthen the flabby areas. Sarvangasana, halasana, bhujangasana, salabhasana, dhanurasana, chakrasana, naukasana, ardha matsyendrasana, paschimottanasana, vajrasana, yogamudra and trikonasana are recommended. Yogic kriyas like kunjal and jalneti and pranayamas such as kapalbhati and bhastrika are also helpful in normalising body weight. The patient should also adopt measures which bring on excessive perspiration such as sauna baths, steam bath and heavy massage. They help to reduce weight. Above all, obese persons should make every effort to avoid negative motions such as anxiety, fear, hostility and insecurity and develop a positive outlook on life.

Chapter 77

Peptic Ulcer

In the natural cure of peptic ulcer, diet is of supreme importance. The diet should be so arranged as to supply adequate nutrition to afford rest to the disturbed organs, to maintain continuous neutralisation of the gastric acid, to inhibit production of acid and to lessen mechanical and chemical irritation. Milk, cream, butter, fruits, and fresh, raw and boiled vegetables, natural foods and natural vitamin supplements are the best diet for an ulcer patient. The most effective remedy for peptic ulcers is bananas. Bananas neutralises the over acidity of the gastric juices and reduces the irritation of the ulcer by quoting the lining of the stomach. Banana and milk are considered an ideal diet for the patients who are in an advanced state of the disease.

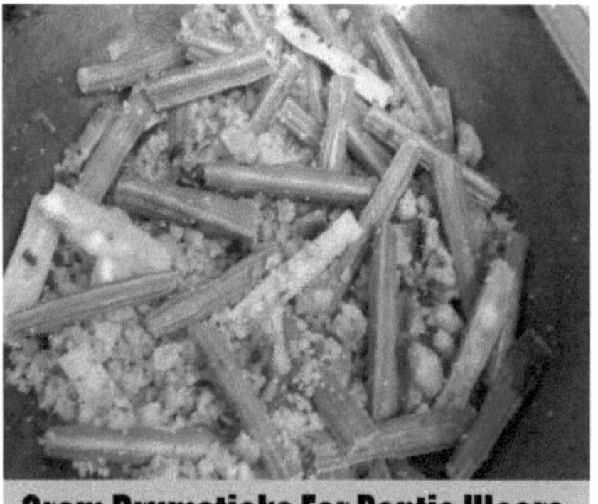

Gram Drumsticks For Peptic Ulcers

Almond milk made from blanched almonds in a blender is very advantageous as it binds the surplus of acid in the stomach and supplies high quality proteins. Raw goat's milk is also extremely beneficial. Cabbage is regarded as another useful home remedy for peptic ulcers. The leaves of kalyana murangal tree, which is a variety of drumstick found in South India, have also proved helpful in the curing of the ulcers. The leaves of this tree are ground into a paste and taken mixed with yogurt daily. Raw vegetables juices, mainly carrot and cabbage juices are beneficial in the treatment of the peptic ulcers. Carrot juice may be taken either alone or in combination with spinach or beat and cucumber.

An ulcer patient, should never eat when tired or emotionally upset, nor when he is not hungry even if it is meal time, nor when his mouth is dry. He should eat only natural foods and take food in as dry a form as possible. Meals must be small and frequent. All foods and drinks which are either too hot or too cold should be avoided. The ulcer patient should drink eight to ten glasses of water every day. However, he should not drink water during or with meals, but only half an hour before or one hour after he has eaten. Alternate hot and cold hip baths for ten to fifteen minutes and a mud pack applied over the lower abdominal for half an hour on a daily basis will help the ulcers to heal. The hip bath or the mud pack should be taken on an empty stomach and should be followed by a walk.

Daily massages and deep breathing exercises also help in the cure of peptic ulcer. Above all, the patient must try to rid himself of worries and stay cheerful. Asanas which are beneficial in the treatment of hyperacidity and ulcers are vajrasana, uttanpadasana, pavana muktasana, bhujangasana, paschimottanasana. Yogic kriyas like jalneti and pranayamas like anuloma-viloma, sitali and sitkari are also beneficial.

Chapter 78

Pyorrhoea

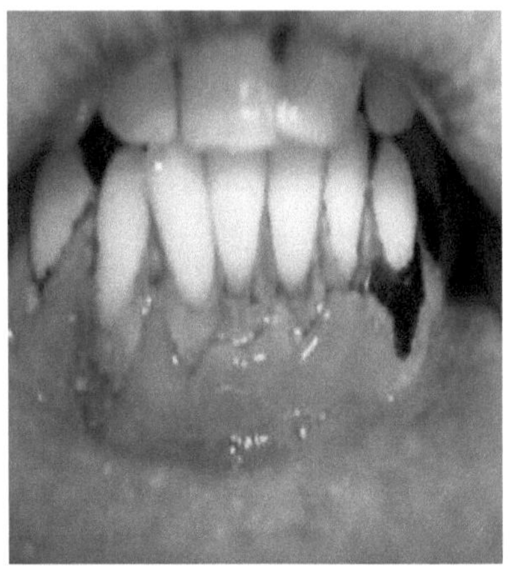

In the natural remedy of pyorrhoea, the patient should commence the treatment with a short juice fast for three to five days. The juice of a fresh orange diluted with water should be taken at two-hourly intervals from 8 a.m. to 8 p.m. during this period. If the orange juice does not agree, carrot juice may be taken. The bowels should be cleansed on a daily basis during this period with a warm water enema. If constipation is habitual, all steps should be taken for its eradication. After the juice fast, the patient should spend a further three to five days on an exclusive fresh fruit diet. In this course of therapy, he should have three meals a day, at five-hourly intervals of fresh juicy fruits such as apples, pears, grapes, grape-fruit, oranges, pineapple and melon.

Subsequently the patient may embark upon a balanced diet, with emphasis on fresh fruits, green salads, whole meal bread, properly cooked vegetables, cheese, nuts, and milk. White bread, white sugar and all refined and tinned foods must be totally given up. Condiments, sauces, alcohol, coffee and strong tea as well as meat and other flesh foods should also be avoided. The patient should also keep away from starchy and sticky foods. The teeth and gum, like other parts of the body require exercise. This can be achieved by eating hard and fibrous foods. Wheat is especially valuable in the prevention and treatment of Pyorrhoea. It takes time to eat wheat chappatis and as it is generally taken with other foods, it compels the chewing of other foods also. This not only provides the needed exercise for the teeth and gum but also a great aid to digestion.

Chewing unripe guava is an excellent tonic for teeth and gums. It stops the bleeding from gums due its styptic effect and richness in vitamin C. Chewing its tender leaves also helps in curing bleeding from gums and keeps the teeth healthy. Lemon and lime are also useful in Pyorrhoea due to their high vitamin C-content. They toughen the gums and teeth and are very useful for preventing and curing acute inflammations of the gum margins. Raw spinach juice is another important food remedy for the prevention and treatment of Pyorrhoea because of its advantageous effect on the teeth and gums. This effect is usually enhanced if the spinach juice is taken in combination with carrot juice. A permanent aid for this problem has been found in the use of natural raw foods and in drinking a sufficient quantity of carrot and spinach juice.

The daily dry friction and hip bath and the breathing and other exercises should form a part of the morning routine. A hot Epsom-salt bath taken twice weekly will also be beneficial. As regards local treatment, the teeth should be cleansed every morning and night with a little lemon juice squeezed on the toothbrush, after it has been dipped into warm water. Afterwards mouth should be well rinsed with warm water containing lemon juice. The forefinger of the right hand should be rubbed gently over the gums for a minute or two after each brushing.

Chapter 79

Influenza

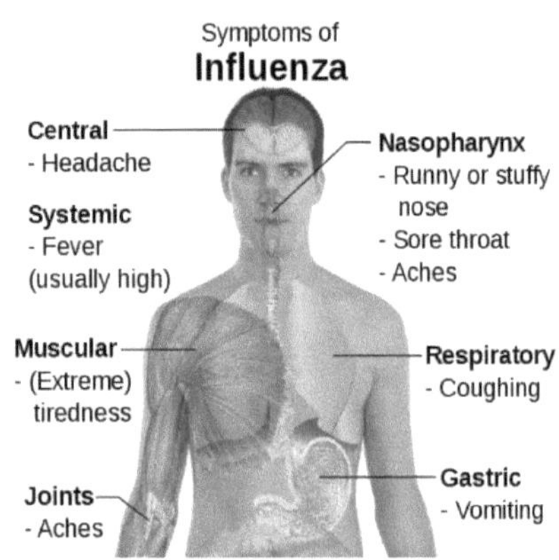

Natural cure of influenza prescribes that the patient should abstain from all solid foods and only drink fruit and vegetable juices diluted with water, depending on the severity of the disease. The juice fast should be continued till the temperature comes down to normal. The warm water enema should be taken on a daily basis during this period to cleanse the bowels. After fever subsides the patient may adopt an all-fruit diet for two or three days. In this regimen, the patient should take three meals a day of fresh juicy fruits such as apples, pears, grapes, oranges, pineapple, peaches and melons at five-hourly intervals. Bananas or dried, stewed or tinned fruits however, should not be taken. No other food stuff should be added to the fruit meals; otherwise the value of the treatment will be lost.

After the fruit diet, the patient may take on a well-balanced diet of three basic food groups namely, (i) seeds, nuts and grains, (ii) vegetables, and (iii) fruits. Spices and condiments, and pickles, which make food more palatal and lead to overeating, must be avoided. Lemon juice may be used in salad dressing. Certain remedies have been found highly advantageous in the treatment of influenza. The most significant of these is the use of long pepper. Half a teaspoonful of the powder of the long pepper with two teaspoonfuls of honey and half a teaspoonful of juice of ginger should be taken thrice a day. This will help to a great extent if taken in initial stages of the disease. It is particularly useful in avoiding complications which follow the onset of the disease, namely, the involvement of the larynx and bronchial tube.

Another excellent medication for influenza is the green leaves of basil or tulsi plant. About one gram of these leaves should be boiled along with some ginger in half a liter of water till about half the water is left. This decoction should be taken as tea. It gives instant relief. Garlic and turmeric are other effective food medicines for influenza. Garlic is useful as a general antiseptic and should be given as much as the patient can bear. Garlic juice may also be sucked up the nose. A teaspoonful of turmeric powder should be mixed in a cup of warm milk and taken three times in the day. It will prevent complications arising from influenza and also activate the liver which becomes sluggish during the attack.

Chapter 80

Stress

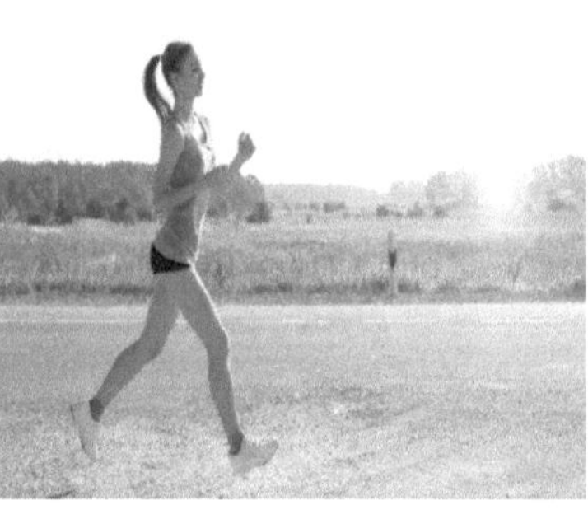

Natural remedy for stress involves a complete alteration in the life style of the patient. His diet should be made of foods which, in combination, would supply all the necessary nutrients. It has been found that a diet which contains liberal quantities of (i) seeds, nuts and grains, (ii) vegetables, and (iii) fruits would give a sufficient amount of all the vital nutrients. Each of these food groups should roughly form the bulk of one of the three meals. These three basic health building foods should be supplemented with certain special foods such as milk, vegetable oils and honey.

There are many foods which are supportive in meeting the demands of stress and should be taken on a regular basis by the patient. These are yogurt, blackstrap molasses, seeds, and sprouts. Yogurt is rich in vitamin A, B complex and D. It relieves insomnia, migraine headache and cramps associated with menstruation. Blackstrap molasses, a by product of sugar refining process, is rich in iron and B vitamins. It guards against anemia and is good for heart diseases. Seeds such as alfalfa, sunflower, and pumpkin and sprouts are rich in calcium and quite of use as deterrents of listlessness and anxiety. Steam cooked vegetables are best as boiling causes many vitamins and minerals to be dispelled into the water. The leaves of holy basil, known as tulsi in the vernacular, are extremely valuable in the healing of stress.

Certain nutrients are beneficial in relieving stress. These are vitamins A and B, minerals such as calcium, potassium and magnesium which diminish the feeling of irritability and anxiety. Vitamin A is found in green and yellow vegetables. Some of the valuable sources of vitamin B are cashews, green leafy vegetables, yeast, sprouts and bananas. An element of vitamin B complex, pantothenic acid is in particular important in preventing stress. It has a deep consequence on the adrenal glands and the immune system and adequate amount of this vitamin along with vitamin A can help prevent many of the changes caused by stress. Potassium deficiencies are associated with breathlessness, fatigue, insomnia and low blood pressure. Potassium is indispensable for healthy heart muscles. Nuts and unrefined grains are good sources of potassium.

Calcium is a natural sedative. Deficiencies can cause fatigue, nervousness and tension. Dairy products, eggs, almonds, and soyabeans are rich sources of calcium. Magnesium is known as nature's tranquiliser and is associated with the prevention of heart attack. Deficiencies may lead to excitability, irritability, apprehension and emotional disorders. Magnesium is also required for absorption of calcium and potassium and is found in many fruits, vegetables, seeds, dates and prunes. There are certain foods which are associated with stress and anxiety and should be scrupulously avoided by patients. These foods are caffeine and many soft drinks, which cause nervousness, irritability and palpitation. Regular physical exercise plays an important role in the fight against stress. Exercise not only keeps the body physically and mentally fit, it also provides amusement and mental respite. One can jog, run, walk or play games, depending upon one's liking. Walking is the simplest and safest exercise. One should take a brisk walk for forty five minutes on a daily basis. Yogic asanas, kriyas and simple pranayamas, beneficial for safeguarding of general health and mental relaxation, can serve as the best shock absorbers against stress. These include asanas like pavana muktasana, sarvagasana, halasana, ardha matsyendrasana, bhujangasana, dhanurasana, yogamudra, padmasana, trikonasana, kriyas like kunjal and jalneti and pranayamas such as kapalbhati, anuloma- viloma, sitali, sitkari and bhramari. Recreation and rest are equally important and patient should set a definite time for spare time activities. They should also take a holiday at regular intervals. And above all, they should simplify their lifestyles to do away with unnecessary stress.

Chapter 81

Tuberculosis

In the natural remedy for tuberculosis, the patient should be put on an exclusive fresh fruit diet for three or four days. He should have three meals a day of fresh, juicy fruits, such as apples, oranges, pineapple, grapes, pears, peaches, melon or any other juicy fruit in season. Bananas, dried or tinned fruits should not be taken. For drinks, unsweetened lemon water or plain water either hot or cold may be taken. After the all fruit diet, the patient should take on a fruit and milk diet. For this diet, the meals are specifically the same as the all fruit diet, but with milk added to each fruit meal.

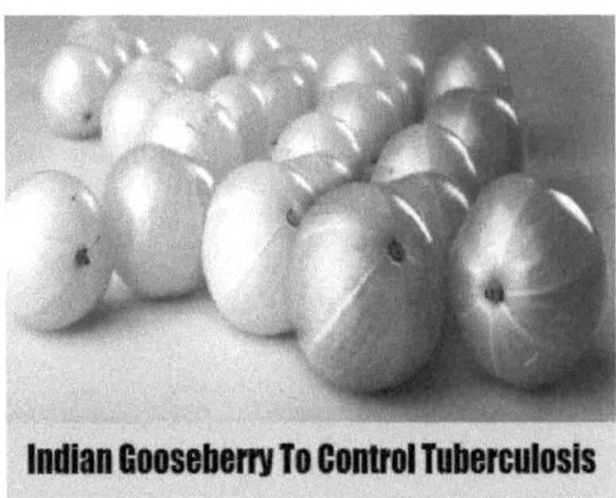

Indian Gooseberry To Control Tuberculosis

The patient may commence with a litre of milk the first day and increase by quarter liter on a daily basis up to two to two and a half litres according to how the milk agrees. The fruit and milk diet should be continued for four to six weeks.

After that, the following dietary may be adopted:

- **Breakfast:** Fresh fruits, as obtainable, and milk. Other dried fruits may also be taken, if desired.
- **Lunch:** Steamed vegetables as obtainable, one or two whole wheat chappatis and a glass of buttermilk.
- **Dinner:** A bowl of raw salad of appropriate vegetables with whole wheat bread and butter. Stewed fruit may be taken for dessert.

The chief remedial agent needed for the cure of tuberculosis is calcium. Milk, being the richest food source for the supply of organic calcium to the body, should be taken abundantly. During the first few days of the treatment, the bowels should be cleansed on a daily basis with the tepid water enema and afterwards as necessary. The patient should avoid all devitalised foods such as white bread, white sugar, refined cereals, puddings and pies, tinned, canned and preserved foods. He should also avoid strong tea, coffee, condiments, pickles, sauces, etc.

The custard apple is regarded as a valuable food remedy for tuberculosis. It is said to have the qualities of rejuvenating drugs. Indian gooseberry has proved to be a successful medication for tuberculosis. A tablespoonful each of fresh amla juice and honey mixed together should be taken every morning in this situation. Its habitual use will promote vigour and liveliness in the body within a few days. Regular use of radish is also advantageous. The patient should take complete rest of both mind and body. Fresh air is always imperative in curing the disease and the patient should spend most of the time in the open air and should sleep in a well ventilated room. Sunshine is also very important as tuber bacilli are rapidly killed by exposure to sun rays. Other beneficial steps towards curing the disease are avoidance of nervous tension, slow massage, deep breathing and light occupation to make sure mental recreation.

Water treatments are helpful in cases of tuberculosis. The patient's fundamental resistance can be built up by a cautiously planned graduated cold bath routine twice a day. The intensity of the cold applications should be gradually increased to achieve satisfactory results. However, care must be taken to keep the patient from catching a cool. A short hot fomentation with alternate short cold application to the chest and back, and in the stomach region or a neutral immersion bath (water temperature 98 O to 100 o F) for an hour just before retiring at night is also advantageous. Certain yogic practices are valuable in the treatment of tuberculosis in its early stages. These include asanas like sarvangasana, Viparita Karani, and shavasana and jalneti kriya and anuloma-viloma pranayama.

Chapter 82

Pre-Menstrual Syndrome

Natural remedy for pre- menstrual syndrome depends on the severity of the symptoms. In case of mild symptoms, the difficulty can be solved by an alteration of routine. Extra work and hectic situation should be avoided. Fluids should be reasonably restricted and care should be taken not to add extra salt to the food. The patient's partner and family members should be educated about all the aspects of the pre-menstrual syndrome. The patient should not take any oral contraceptives as these may cause fluid retention and lowering of the plasma levels. Hormonal discrepancy and infections of the uterus can be helped by a natural diet schedule.

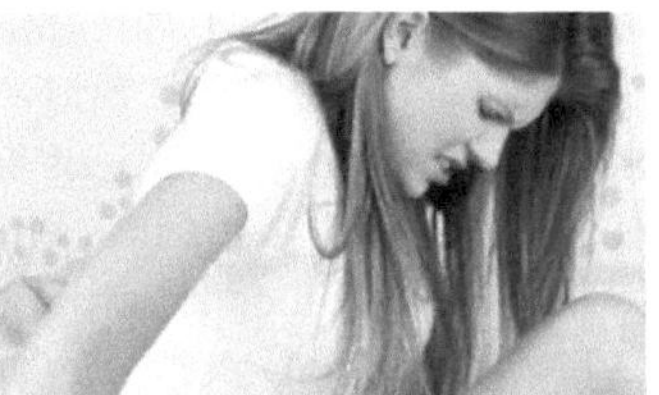

Most women feel tension arising from chronic constipation, so it is necessary to treat this condition first. Constipation can be relieved by a tepid water enema and moderate intake of seasonal fruits and vegetables and simple fibrous meals. Other treatment for the pre-menstrual syndrome includes normal cold hip baths for ten to fifteen minutes twice a day. Tension will also be dissipated with this therapy. Hot foot baths followed by a cold compress to the lower abdomen and the inner surfaces of the thighs also help to ease uterine congestion and tension. If the cold hip bath is not feasible, a wet girdle pack applied twice a day on empty stomach is very advantageous for clearing up uterine congestion and improving bowel function.

Diet pays an imperative role in preventing premenstrual syndrome. The patient should avoid refined sugars, coffee, tea, tobacco, other stimulants, oily or spicy food and all meats. A regular practice of yoga asanas, especially those recommended for strengthening the genito -urinary system will be very functional in overcoming premenstrual syndrome. These asanas are bhujangasana, salabhasana, vajrasana, ardha matsyendrasana, paschimotanasana and trikonasana. Great respite can also be obtained by manipulating the tender points soothingly, on the big as well as other toes of the feet. Other helpful measures are brisk walks and abdominal exercises which are good for intensification the abdominal muscles and pelvic organs. Mental composure is an important factor. Negative mental attitudes like fear, worry, anger, jealousy, nervousness and inferiority complex should be eliminated by positive thinking and meditation.

Chapter 83

Inflammation of Uterus

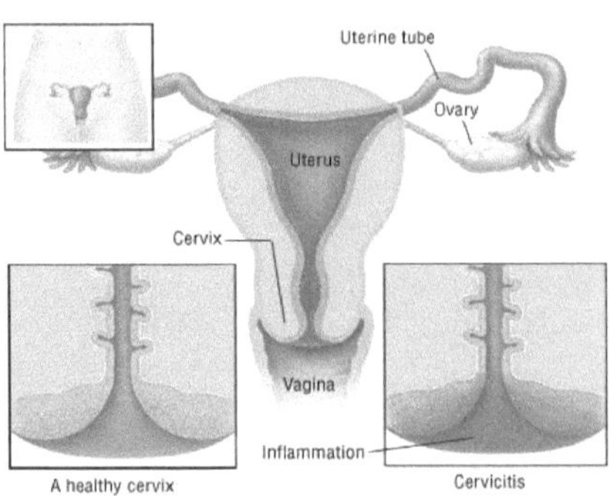

In the natural remedy for the inflammation of the uterus, water therapy is of great help. In case the inflammation is caused by exposure to cold at the time of menstruation, the patient should commence the treatment with a hot leg bath. This may be replaced by hot hip bath after two or three days. In case of pain, hot and cold hip baths will be advantageous. The water should be changed from hot to cold, every two minutes and this should be repeated thrice. This disease produces the propensity towards constipation, so the patient should take an enema once on a daily basis with lukewarm water as can be at ease borne by the patient. It is also wise to apply alternate compress on the abdomen just before employing enema.

In the chronic form the cure should aim at increasing the general vitality. Initially the patient should resort to fasting on orange juice and water for two or three days. The course of action is to take every two hours from 8 a.m. to 8 p.m. the juice of an orange diluted with warm water. If the orange juice does not agree, juices of vegetable such as carrots and cucumber may be taken. A warm water enema may be taken each day while fasting to cleanse the bowels. After the short juice fast, the patient may assume an all-fruit diet for about two days, taking three meals a day of fresh juicy fruits such as apples, orange, pineapple, pears, grapes, grapefruit, peaches and melon. After the juice fast the patient should follow a well balanced diet of seeds, nuts, and grains, vegetables and fruits. This diet should be supplemented with milk, vegetable oil, yogurt, butter-milk and honey.

A further short juice fast or periods on the all-fruit diet may be required at intervals of a month or two, according to the needs of the case. If constipation is regular, all steps should be taken for its eradication. White flour products, sugar, confectionery, rich cakes, pastries, sweets, refined cereals, tinned or preserved foods, flesh foods, rich, heavy and greasy foods, pickles, condiments, and sauces should be avoided. The patient should also embark on moderate exercise and walking in fresh air as it will add to general health and vitality. Yogic asanas such as bhujangasana, sarvangasana, uttanasana, and shavasana are also advantageous in the treatment of inflammation of the uterus.

Chapter 84

Pruritus Vulvae

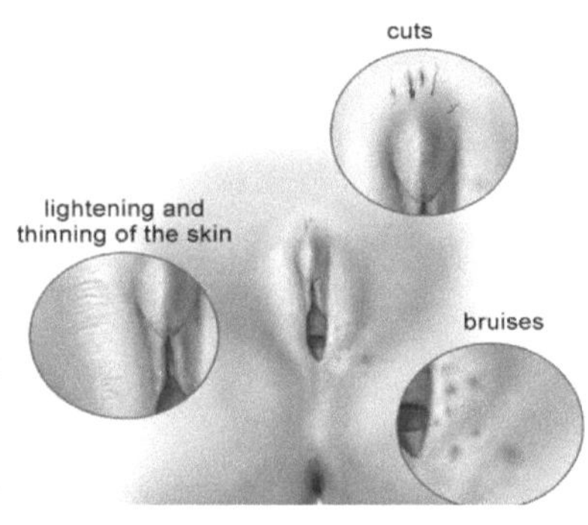

Natural remedy for pruritus vulvae depends on two fundamental principles, namely, to get rid of any underlying cause and to stop further damage to the skin by scratching or by inappropriate application. The most vital aspect in the treatment of pruritus vulvae caused by infections through fungus or parasites is cleanliness. Bowels should be kept clean either through enemas or a natural diet. The patient must wear clean clothes to stay away from this problem. After urination, the vagina should be carefully washed with plain cold water. In case of severe pruritus, it is wise to wash the vulva with neem leaves decoction and apply green light charged coconut oil.

Treatments like neem water vaginal douches help kill bacteria and fungus. The affect reaction should be exposed to green coloured light or rays of the sun through green coloured glass for twenty five to thirty minutes. This will help lessen infections. Pruritus vulvae resulting from discharges from the uterus, cervix or vagina causes inflammations. This can be reduced by usual application of mud packs on the lower abdomen, twice or thrice on a daily basis. A cold hip bath may also be taken for ten minutes. An alternate hot and cold hip bath is particularly useful in reducing inflammation. In cases of pruritus resulting from diabetes mellitus, jaundice, glycosuria, uraemia and other toxic states, specific diets and treatments for these complaints should be followed before Pruritus could be cured. Skin diseases like psoriasis, scabies, and fungal infections should be treated through nature cure methods. These include steam baths, mud baths, immersion baths, sun baths, spine baths and colour therapy.

Diet plays a significant role in the treatment of pruritus vulvae. In the beginning the patient should be put on a juice fast for a few days. She should drink fruit and vegetable juices, diluted with water. A lukewarm water enema should be used on a daily basis during the period of fasting to cleanse the bowels. Fasting helps relieve the toxic conditions not in just the affected region but also the whole body. Thus inflammation is reduced. The diet after the juice fast could comprise seasonal fruits, vegetables, salads, sprouts, soups or buttermilk. Cooked food should be included in the diet only much later. The patient should avoid all processed, refined and denatured foods such as white sugar, white flour and all products made from them as well as coffee, tea, eggs, meat, spicy and oily foods. Alcohol and smoking are to be entirely eliminated. A natural mode of life will go a long way in overcoming pruritus vulvae. It will also lead to enhancement in health in general.

RAPIDEX ENGLISH SPEAKING COURSE/EXCEL ENGLISH SPEAKING COURSE

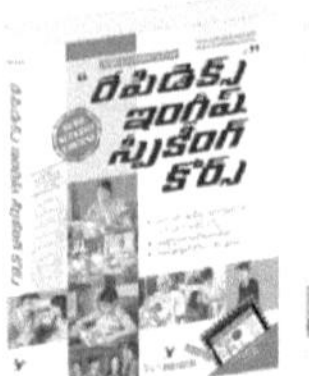
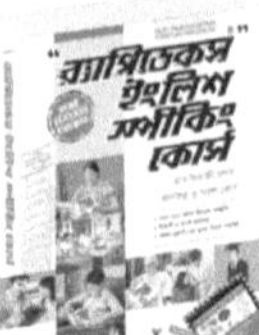
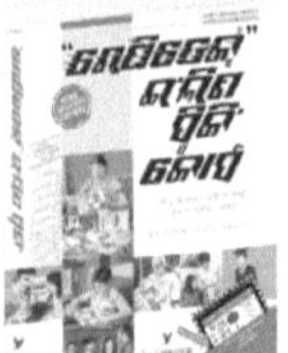
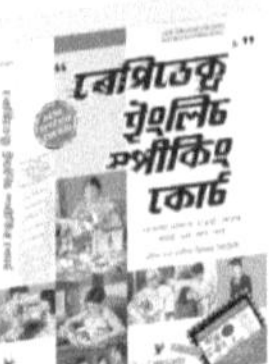
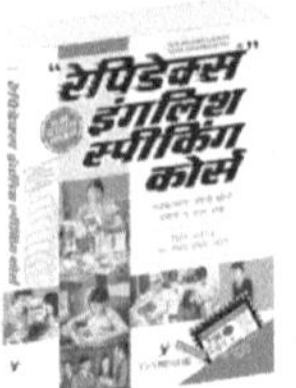

ISBN : 9789381448908 (Telugu)

ISBN : 9789381448915 (Bangla)

ISBN : 9789381448922 (Oriya)

ISBN : 9789381448939 (Assamese)

ISBN : 9789381448946 (Nepalese)

Published in sixteen languages
Hindi, Malayalam, Tamil, Telugu, Kannada, Marathi, Gujarati, Bangla, Oriya, Urdu, Assamese, Punjabi, Nepalese, Persian, Arabic and Sinhalese

REGIONAL LANGUAGE/SPOKEN ENGLISH/LEARNING COURSES

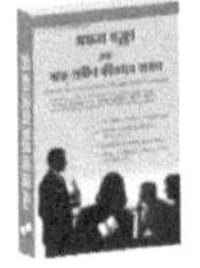
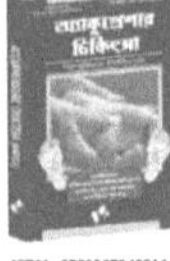
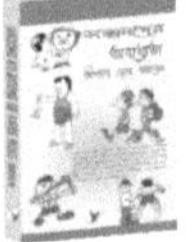
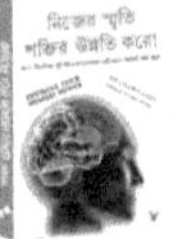
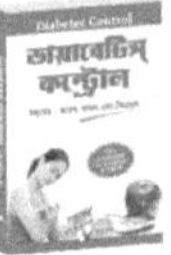
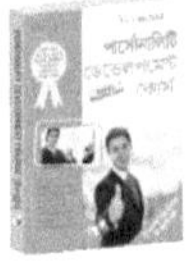
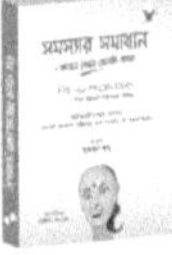
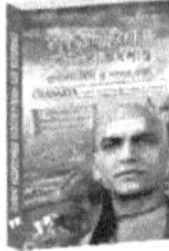

ISBN : 9789357940054 (Bangla)

ISBN : 9789357940016 (Bangla)

ISBN :9789357940023 (Bangla)

ISBN : 9789357940085 (Bangla)

ISBN : 9789357940825 (Bangla)

ISBN : 9789357940092 (Bangla)

ISBN : 9789357940009 (Bangla)

ISBN : 9789357940030 (Bangla)

ISBN : 9789357941303 *(2 Colour Book)*

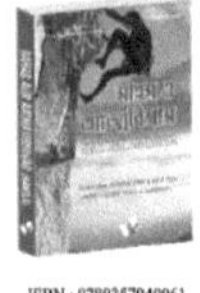
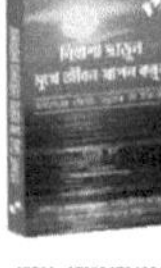
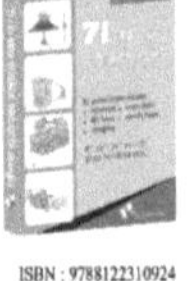
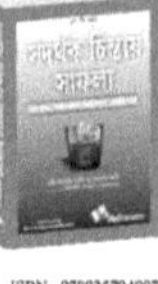
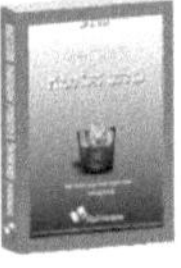
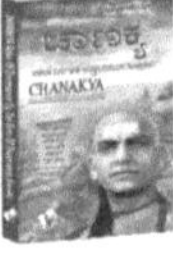
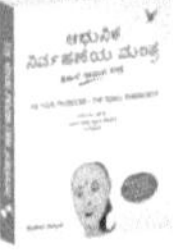
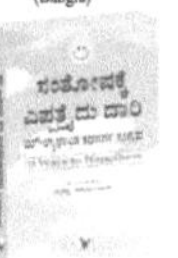

ISBN : 9789357940061 (Bangla)

ISBN : 9789357940047 (Bangla)

ISBN : 9788122310924 (Bangla)

ISBN : 9789357940078 (Bangla)

ISBN 9789350570357 (Kannada)

ISBN : 9789350571200 (Kannada)

ISBN : 9789350570340 (Kannada)

ISBN : 9789350570944 (Kannada)

(Coming Soon) Marathi

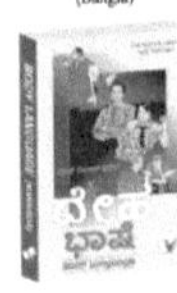
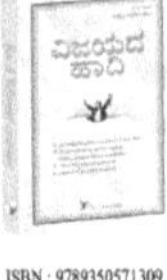
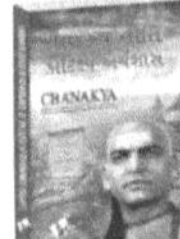
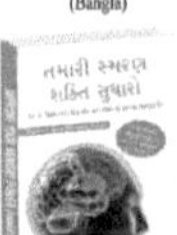
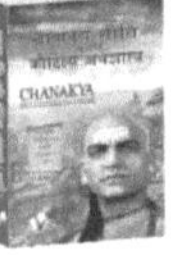
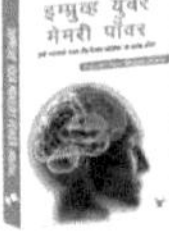
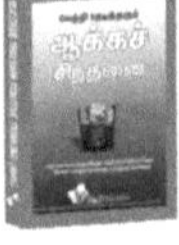
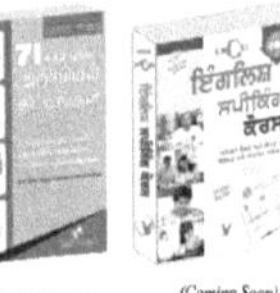

ISBN : 9789350570951 (Kannada)

ISBN : 9789350571309 (Kannada)

ISBN : 9789350571828 (Gujarati)

ISBN : 9789350571781 (Gujarati)

ISBN : 9789350571811 (Marathi)

ISBN : 9789350571804 (Marathi)

ISBN : 9789381384138 (Tamil)

ISBN : 9789381384121 (Tamil)

(Coming Soon) Punjabi

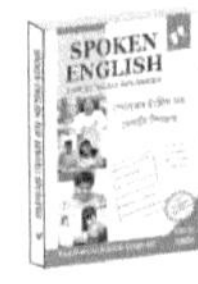
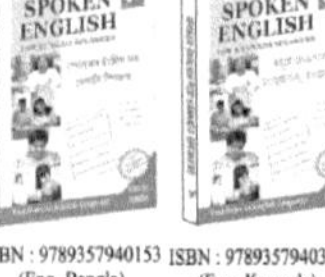
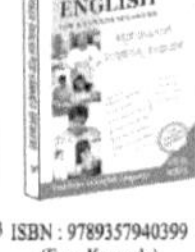

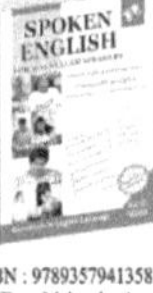
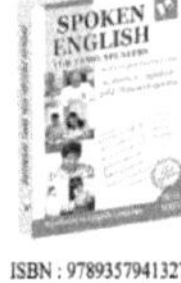

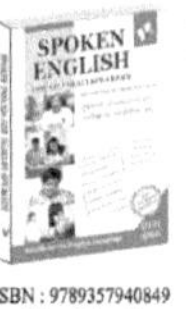
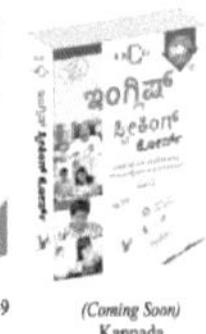

ISBN : 9789357940153 (Eng.-Bangla)

ISBN : 9789357940399 (Eng.-Kannada)

ISBN : 9789357940375 (Eng.-Odia)

ISBN : 9789357940382 (Eng.-Telugu)

ISBN : 9789357941358 (Eng.-Malayalam)

ISBN : 9789357941327 (Eng.-Tamil)

ISBN : 9789357940856 (Eng.-Marathi)

ISBN : 9789357940849 (Eng.-Gujarati)

(Coming Soon) Kannada

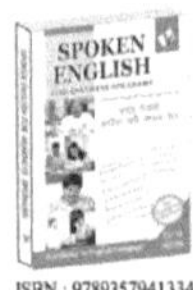
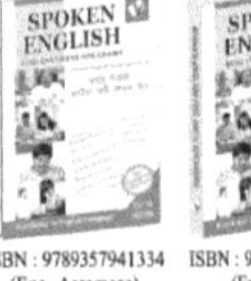
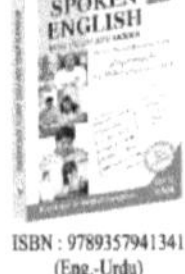
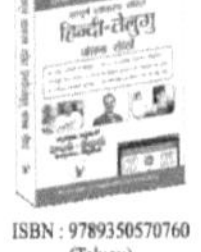
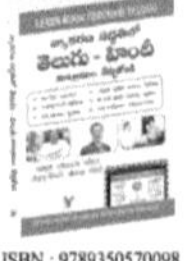
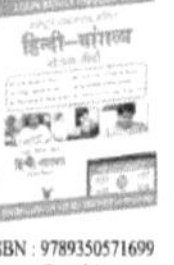
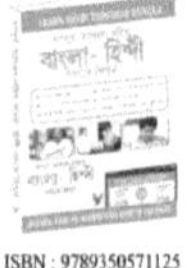
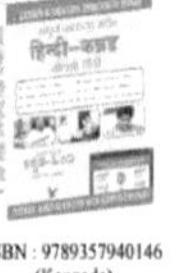
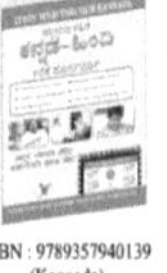

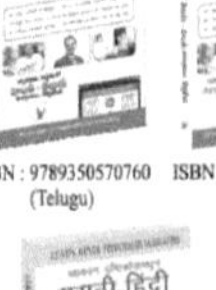

ISBN : 9789357941334 (Eng.-Assamese)

ISBN : 9789357941341 (Eng.-Urdu)

ISBN : 9789350570760 (Telugu)

ISBN : 9789350570098 (Telugu)

ISBN : 9789350571699 (Bangla)

ISBN : 9789350571125 (Bangla)

ISBN : 9789357940146 (Kannada)

ISBN : 9789357940139 (Kannada)

(Coming Soon) Gujarati

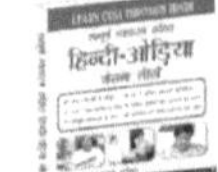
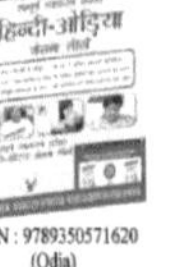
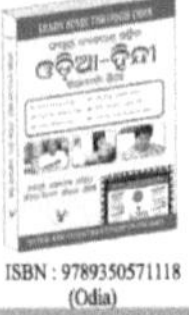
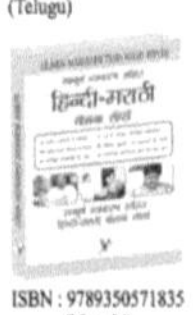
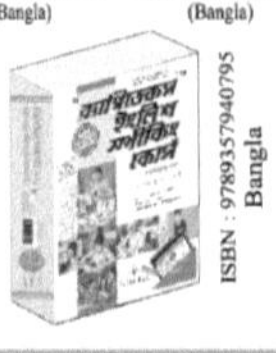
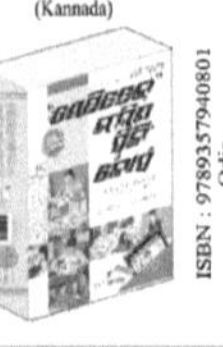

ISBN : 9789350571620 (Odia)

ISBN : 9789350571118 (Odia)

ISBN : 9789350570982 (Marathi)

ISBN : 9789350571835 (Marathi)

ISBN : 9789357940795 Bangla

ISBN : 9789357940801 Odia

ISBN : 9789357940818 Telugu

All Books Available on Flipkart, Amazon, Infibeam, Snapdeal, Shopcluse • marketing@vspublishers.com

CAREER & BUSINESS/SELF-HELP/PERSONALITY DEVELOPMENT/STRESS MANAGEMENT

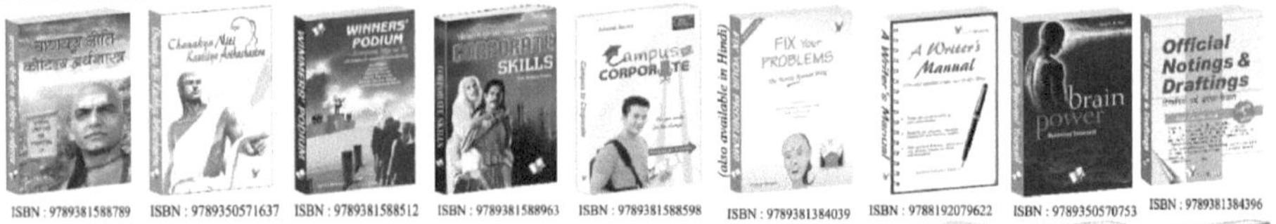

ISBN : 9789381588789 ISBN : 9789350571637 ISBN : 9789381588512 ISBN : 9789381588963 ISBN : 9789381588598 ISBN : 9789381384039 ISBN : 9788192079622 ISBN : 9789350570753 ISBN : 9789381384396

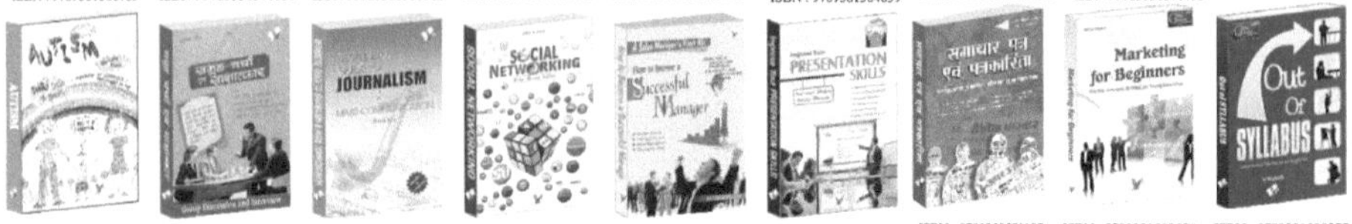

ISBN : 9789381384541 ISBN : 9789350570968 ISBN : 9789381384527 ISBN : 9789381588666 ISBN : 9789381384541 ISBN : 9789381384107 ISBN : 9789350571187 ISBN : 9789381588574 ISBN : 9789381588277

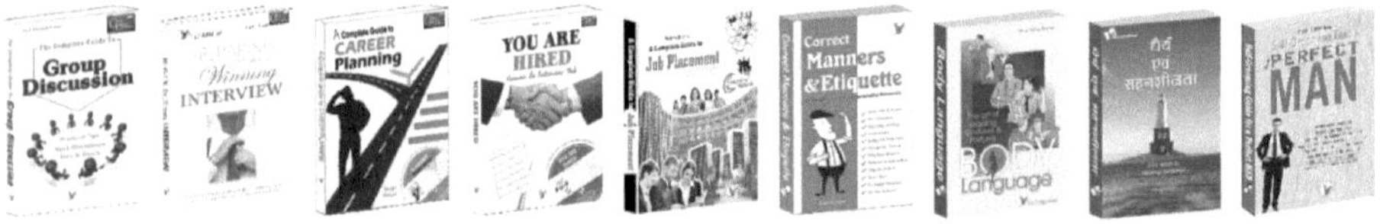

ISBN : 9789381588222 ISBN : 9789381384213 ISBN : 9789381588772 ISBN : 9789381588949 ISBN : 9789357940108 ISBN : 9789381384152 ISBN : 9789381384145 ISBN : 9789381448564 ISBN : 9789381384473

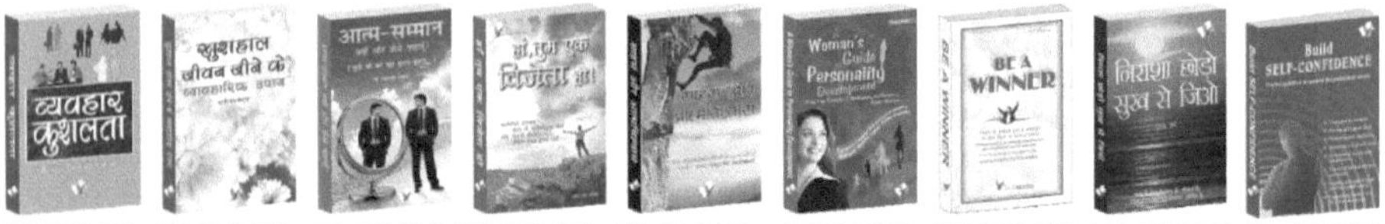

ISBN : 9789381448595 ISBN : 9789381448670 ISBN : 9789381588253 ISBN : 9789381448755 ISBN : 9789381448649 ISBN : 9789381384480 ISBN : 9789350571309 ISBN : 9789381448632 ISBN : 9789381384893

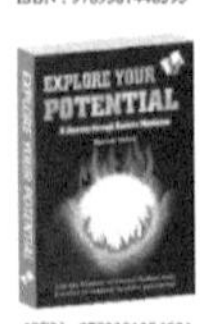
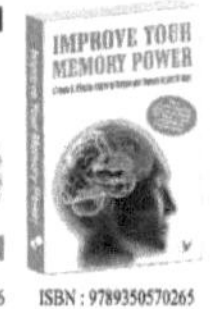
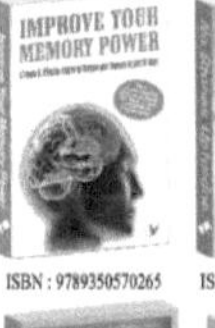
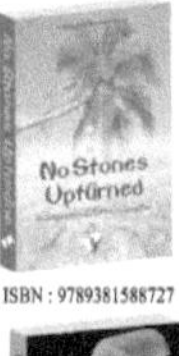
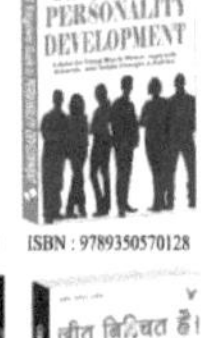
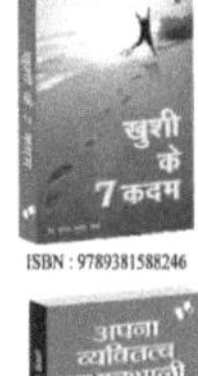
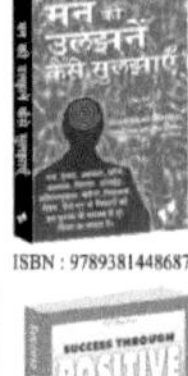
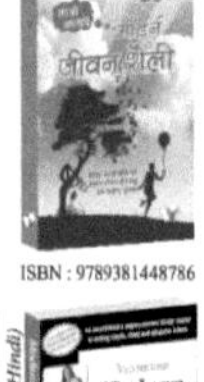
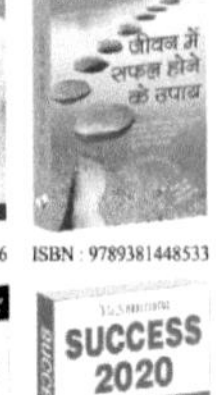

ISBN : 9789381384091 ISBN : 9789381384176 ISBN : 9789350570265 ISBN : 9789381588727 ISBN : 9789350570128 ISBN : 9789381588246 ISBN : 9789381448687 ISBN : 9789381448786 ISBN : 9789381448533

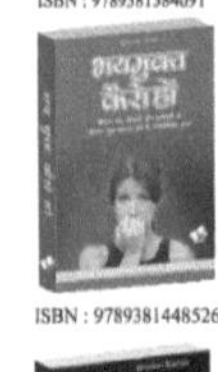
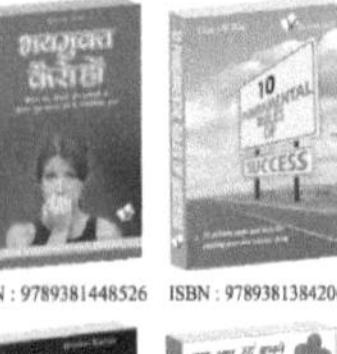
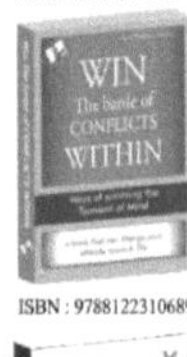
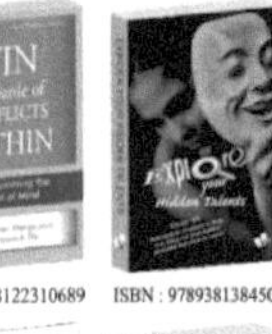
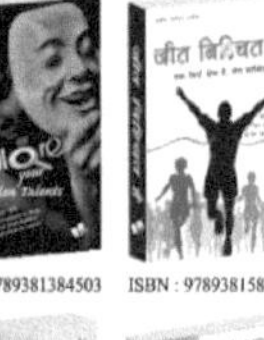
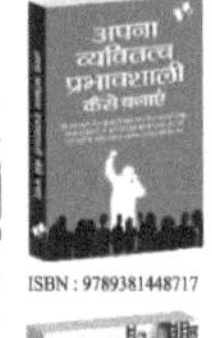
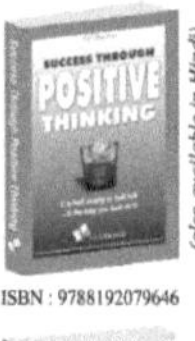
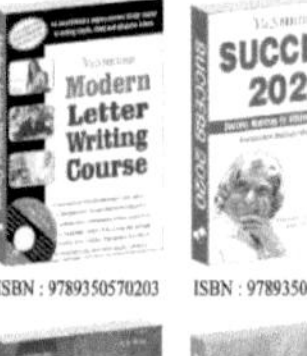

ISBN : 9789381448526 ISBN : 9789381384206 ISBN : 9788122310689 ISBN : 9789381384503 ISBN : 9789381588505 ISBN : 9789381448717 ISBN : 9788192079646 ISBN : 9789350570203 ISBN : 9789350570272

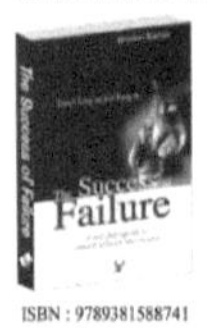
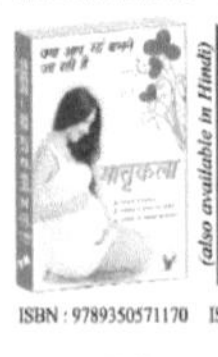
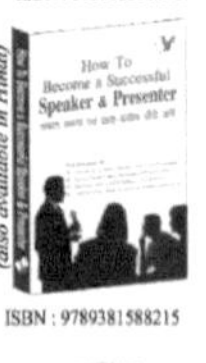
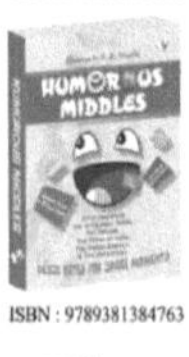
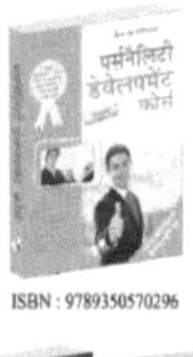
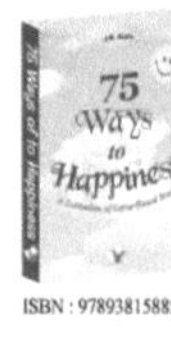
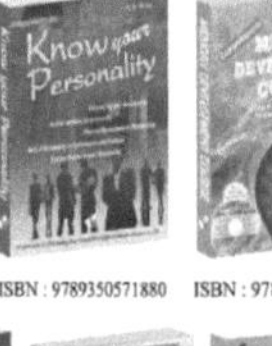
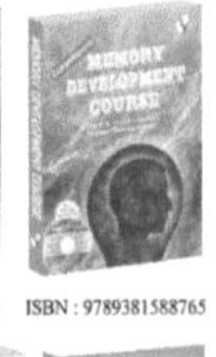

ISBN : 9789381588741 ISBN : 9789350571170 ISBN : 9789381588215 ISBN : 9789381384763 ISBN : 9789350570296 ISBN : 9789381588284 ISBN : 9789381588543 ISBN : 9789350571880 ISBN : 9789381588765

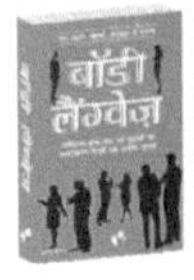
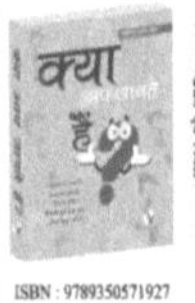
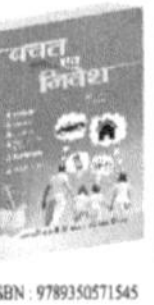
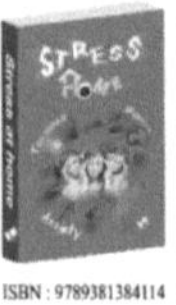
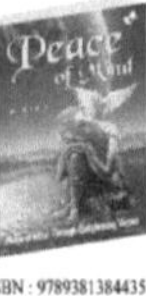
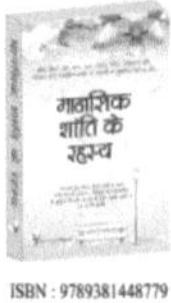
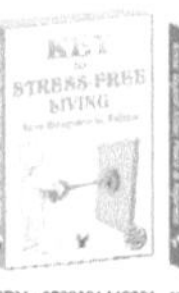
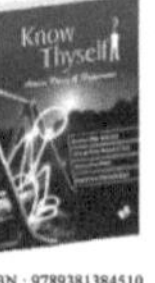
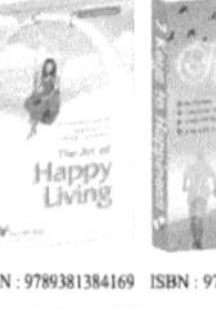

ISBN : 9789350570579 ISBN : 9789350571927 ISBN : 9789350571545 ISBN : 9789381384114 ISBN : 9789381384435 ISBN : 9789381448779 ISBN : 9789381448991 ISBN : 9789381384510 ISBN : 9789381384169 ISBN : 9789350570623

All Books Available on Flipkart, Amazon, Infibeam, Snapdeal, Shopcluse • marketing@vspublishers.com

Printed by Libri Plureos GmbH in Hamburg,
Germany